The Vitamin, Mineral and Herb Guide

A quick overview of the benefits and uses of vitamins, minerals and herbs

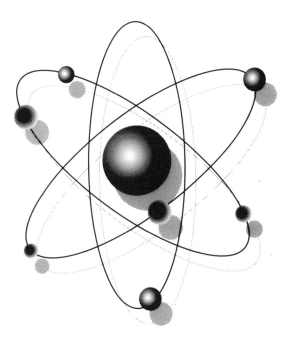

by Russell G. Merrill

This book is intended to serve as a general reference only, and should not be used to replace the advice of a physician. The author and publisher expressly disclaim responsibility for any adverse effects or unforeseen consequences of the applications, preparations, or recommendations contained in this book.

The Vitamin, Mineral and Herb Guide

By Russell G. Merrill

Published by A.R.M. Publications, L.L.C.

Copyright © 1997 by Russell G. Merrill. All rights reserved. Printed in the United States of America. Except as permitted under the United States Copyright Act of 1976. This Vitamin, Mineral and Herb Guide may not be reproduced published, or transmitted, in whole or in part, in any form or by any means, electronic or mechanical, including photocopying, recording or information storage or retrieval system, without the prior written permission of Russell G. Merrill, Post Office Box 12843 La Jolla, California 92039-2843. email: merrillr@adnc.com

Library of Congress Cataloging-in Publication Data

Merrill, R.G.

(The Vitamin, Mineral and Herb Guide)

PRINTED & BOUND IN THE UNITED STATES

10 9 8 7 6 5 4 3 2 1

ISBN:0-9661633-0-3

Single copies may be ordered from A.R.M. Publishers, L.L.C. Post Office Box 12843 La Jolla, CA 92039-2843 USA. Telephone (619) 622-1996 or Fax (619) 622-1992. Quantity discounts are also available. Orders must be on letterhead and include information concerning the intended use of the books and the number of books you wish to purchase.

Acknowledgments

To all of my friends and to the health & nutritional professionals in appreciation for their assistance and support in making this book come to reality.

Editing: Ms. Kathy Mills and Ms. Sue Prelozni
Cover design, graphic design, artwork: Mr. Steve Jurak
Cover photography: Mr. Sam Marsh
Herb photographs: The Lloyd Library and Museum in Cincinnati, Ohio

Thanks also to the American Medical Association, the American Pharmaceutical Association; the American Journal of Chinese Medicine; the American Journal of Clinical Nutrition; the American Journal of Public Heath; the Canadian Pharmaceutical Journal; the Food and Cosmetic Toxicology; the Heath Food Business; the HerbalGram; the International Journal of Sport Nutrition; the Journal of the American College Nutrition; the Journal of the American Dietetics Association: the Journal of the American Medical Technology; the Journal of Biosocial Sciences; the Journal of Natural Products; the Journal of Nutrition; the Journal of Nutritional Biochemistry; the Journal of New Chinese Medicine; the Lancet; the New England Journal of Medicine; the New York Times; Nutritional research; the Reader's Digest Magic and Medicine of Plants; the World Review of Nutrition and Dietetics; Deepak Chopra's Infinite Possibilities for the Body, Mind and Soul; Environmental Nutrition; the Harvard Health Letter; Heath After 50; Health News; Health & Nutrition Letter; the Mayo Clinic Health Letter, the Lifetime Health Letter, the Nutrition Action Health Letter, Dr Andrew Weil's-Self Healing and the Wellness Letter.

Table of Contents

HERBS:

WATER:

BIBLIOGRAPHY:

The Vitamin, Mineral and Herb Guide

1. Introduction to Nutritional Factors.

In the Nutritional Beginning.

The body is a chemical burning oven that generates energy for mental and physical functions. This was first realized from Egyptian pictographs, Circa BC 1500, which offered dietary cures for a variety of afflictions and diseases. The Old Testament also contains numerous records of "laws" for the selection, preparation and storage of foods.

Up to the 1700's.

Hippocrates, born BC 460, was known as "The Father of Medicine". He emphasized the role of diet in the control of disease. Although most of his teachings were without scientific foundation, they did set the medical precedent in considering nutritional factors. In the early 1700's, Rene' de Re'aumur was given credit for his pioneering investigations into the chemical nature of digestion. Antoine Laurent Lavoisier, in the mid 1700's, established the basis for the scientific study of energy metabolism in laboratory animals. During the same period, Dr. James Lind showed the effect of consuming citrus fruits on the treatment and prevention of scurvy. Dr. Lind worked with British sailors to treat and prevent scurvy. Hence came the name "Limeys" for British sailors.

Through the 1800's.

In the early 1800's, researchers from Switzerland and France determined the dietary importance of calcium in dental and bone growth and for health. And in 1838, a chemist from Sweden, Berzelius, determined the role of iron in hemoglobin formation and opened the field of dietary therapy for anemia. At about the same time period, J. B. Boussingault proposed that iodine could be used to prevent goiter, which was based on an observed relationship between diet and the incidence of the disease in South America. In 1862, the first large experimental chamber to study human heat production and oxygen/carbon dioxide exchange was constructed in Germany. With these chambers, scientists were able to prove the law of the conservation of energy for higher animals. Justus von Liebig, in the mid 1800's, developed analytical methods for determining the composition of foods, body tissue and excrement. Carl von Voit, a student of Justus von Liebig, studied the influence of nitrogen on protein metabolism. P. Eijkmann of the Netherlands, demonstrated that beriberi could be induced or cured by dietary substitution of processed or unmilled rice in 1897.

Rapid Advances in the 1990's.

In the first decade of the 1900's, an Englishman, J. G. Hopkins determined that laboratory animals required more than proteins, carbohydrates, fats and salts to sustain life. In 1911, Dr. Casimir Funk named the missing nutritional factor - Vitamine. Dr. Funk was a Polish chemist working at the Lister Institute in London. He derived the word "**vitamine**" from "**vita**" meaning "**life**", and "**amine**", referring to a class of nitrogen-containing organic compounds. It was learned, some time later, that not all vitamins were amines, so the final "**e**" was dropped from the word "**vitamin**".

In the 1920's, researchers from Yale University and the University of Wisconsin isolated vitamin A. The isolation of vitamin A was accomplished by scientifically controlling the diet of laboratory animals. Later on in the mid 1930's, Rudolf Schoenheimer of Columbia University used hydrogen isotopes in tracing metabolic reactions to aid in the identification of several other nutrients. Since the first identification of vitamins in 1911, scientists have identified thirteen (13) vitamins, the last being B12 in the 1940's.

A major discovery was made in 1953 - the discovery of the DNA structure and function. The field of genetics was revolutionized. Francis H. C. Crick and James D. Watson greatly advanced nutritional studies with the explanation of DNA's double-helix structure and the process of its replication.

Since that major discovery, the number and importance of nutritional discoveries per month in the 1980's corresponds to the advances in research that equals the rest of the centuries previous collective discovery. Nutrition research today involves tools and techniques that did not exist a decade ago. Many researchers agree that the total human knowledge about nutrition is estimated to double every two (2) years. The science of nutrition has grown dramatically - it is no longer a single field. Nutritional research is a study of genetics, molecular biology, psychobiology, immunology, pharmacology, neuroscientific research and other scientific fields.

Current Trends.

It has been approximately eighty six (86) years since the "**identification**" of the first vitamin. Today, the rate of laboratory and clinical findings is so great that an individual would have to keep abreast of the findings of the last couple of years in order to be somewhat nutritionally aware. New findings and benefits of vitamins, minerals and herbs for proper nutrition are continuing at a rapid pace.

2. Nutrients.

Nutrients are more than just vitamins and minerals. There are two (2) main categories of Nutrients, **Macronutrients and Micronutrients.** Macronutrients and micronutrients are made up of six (6) important nutrients: Carbohydrates, proteins, fats, minerals, vitamins and water. "**Essential**" nutrients are those nutrients which are necessary for the body to function effectively, and which are not synthesized in the body. These "**essential**" nutrients are necessary for energy, organ function, food utilization and cell growth. The following is a brief description of those nutrients.

2A. Macronutrients.

Macronutrients derived the name because they comprise the greatest portion of the human diet. They are the primary source of energy to the body. Macronutrients supply fuel for work and help to regulate the body's heat. The term, "**calorie (calories)**" signifies the amount of energy that could be released as heat when food is metabolized. Foods that are high in calories are usually high in "**energy value**" and foods that are low in calories are normally low in "**energy value**". The macronutrients are carbohydrates, fats (lipids) and proteins.

Carbohydrates. There are three (3) main types of carbohydrate groups: (1) Monosaccharides, which consists of glucose, galactose and fructose, (2) Disaccharide's, which consists of sucrose, lactose and maltose and (3) Polysaccharides, which consists of starch and cellulose. The sugars are the monosaccharides and disaccharides. The starches are the polysaccharides. Sugars and starches serve as the body's main source of energy. They also help to regulate the metabolism of proteins and fats (lipids). Sugars aid in muscular exertion and contractions. Foods that contain all three (3), sugar, starch and cellulose are known as "**complex**" carbohydrates, an example would be cereals and vegetables.

Carbohydrates are necessary for the digestion and assimilation of other foods. They can be manufactured in the body. One of the sugars, glucose, can be used directly by the cells. Glucose known as "**blood sugar**", is a major component of the blood. Complex sugars, such as, disaccharides and starches are metabolized in the body to form glucose and fructose. They are also used as fuel for the body.

The concentration of glucose in the blood is normally kept within narrow limits. A high concentration of glucose in the blood is known as "**hyperglycemia**", and a low concentration of glucose in the blood is known as "**hypoglycemia**". There are several hormones in the body which keep the **"blood sugar"** within these narrow limits. They are insulin, glucagon, epinephrine, corticosteroids and growth hormones. Some of the sugars in the body are converted to glycogen and are mainly stored in the liver and muscles. The excess is converted to fat and stored throughout the body. Fat cannot be converted to glucose, but can be burned as fuel to save glucose.

Fiber (or cellulose) is another type of carbohydrate. Fiber is found in the skin of fruits, vegetables and grains. A few good sources of fiber are whole-grain breads, peanuts, celery, raisins, green beans, prunes and bran. Fiber serves to facilitate digestion and passes through the intestines substantially unchanged. It has little energy producing potential.

There is scientific evidence that the **"B"** vitamins must be present for proper metabolism of carbohydrates. The total amount of carbohydrates needed by the body depends on a great many factors. Some of which are the person's age, sex, metabolism, the amount of physical activity and the person's weight. It is estimated an individual's diet should contain between 40% and 50% complex carbohydrates.

Proteins. Proteins are the most plentiful substances in the body after water. They are the main structural components of tissues and organs. Proteins are extremely important for maintaining good health, vitality and proper growth and development of all body tissues. They are also vital to the formation of hormones, enzymes and antibodies. Proteins play an important role in rebuilding body tissues and regulating the body's metabolism. There are two (2) types of proteins, fibrous and globular. Fibrous proteins are insoluble and form the structural basis of many body tissues, such as hair, skin, muscles, tendons and cartilage. Globular proteins are soluble and include all enzymes, several hormones (i.e. growth hormones), and various proteins in the blood (i.e. hemoglobin and antibodies). Enzymes and antibodies are formed from proteins. These antibodies help fight off foreign substances.

Proteins consist of larger molecules that are broken down into amino acids during digestion. There are approximately twenty-two (22) amino acids in the body. Fourteen (14) amino acids are manufactured in the body and eight (8) are obtained from a balanced diet. All of the **"essential"** amino acids must be present simultaneously, and in the proper proportions for the body to properly synthesize proteins. Amino acids are necessary for the construction of body proteins and are vital for the growth and maintenance of muscles, blood, internal organs, skin, hair and nails.

There are "**complete**" and "**incomplete**" protein foods. "**Complete**" protein foods are foods that contain all the essential amino acids. "**Incomplete**" protein foods are foods that are low in essential amino acids or lack any one (1) essential amino acid. Meats and dairy products are considered "**complete**" protein foods. Most fruits and vegetables are considered "**incomplete**" protein food. An individual should select well-balanced food groups to obtain all the essential amino acids in their diet. Food supplements may be necessary for an individual to achieve the proper amino acid and/or vitamin and mineral balance.

Protein requirements will differ substantially in each individual. It depends on the individuals age, sex, body size, physical activity level, living habits and different types of stressful conditions, physical and mental. It is therefore, very difficult to determine the optimum daily protein requirement. As a general rule, the National Research Council recommends 0.42 grams of protein per day be consumed for each pound of body weight. This value will vary depending on the daily amino acid intake of an individual.

Fats or Lipids. Fats are the most concentrated energy source in a person's diet. The sources of fats are from animal and plant foods. Fats are oxidized and supply the body with twice as many calories per gram than carbohydrates or proteins. Fats are the carriers for fat-soluble vitamins (A, D, E, and K) and serve to control the rate of digestion in the stomach. Fats slow down the secretions of hydrochloric acid in the stomach, which prolongs the digestion process. They aid in the absorption of vitamin D and helps make calcium available to body tissues, particularly the teeth and bones. Fats are extremely important in the overall function of the body. They protect and hold organs in place, insulate the body from environmental temperature variations and preserves body heat.

Fats consist of two (2) types of fatty acids: "**saturated**" and "**unsaturated**". There are over forty (40) different fatty acids found in nature. "**Saturated**" fatty acids come mainly from animal products and are normally hard at room temperature. "**Unsaturated**" fatty acids come mainly from vegetables, nuts and seeds and are normally liquid at room temperature. A few other sources of fats are milk, eggs and cheese.

There are three (3) essential fatty acids, arachidonic, linoleic and linolenic. Collectively they are known as unsaturated fatty acids. Arachidonic and linolenic acids are necessary for normal growth and the healthy development of blood, blood vessels and nerves. They also play a significant role in maintaining healthy skin and tissues. Arachidonic and linolenic acids can be synthesized in the body from linoleic acid. Linoleic acid is an "**essential**" fatty acid - meaning it cannot be synthesized from macronutrients. It is supplied through a person's diet or through food supplements. There is no specific required "**amount**" of fat required in a person's diet. An individual should consume approximately 15% of their caloric intake as fat. This will insure the absorption of fat-soluble vitamins and linoleic acid.

Cholesterol is a fat-related substance called a "**lipid**". It is a necessary component for good health. Cholesterol is found in most body tissues, including the brain, blood cells, liver and the nervous system. The liver makes most cholesterol in the blood with some being absorbed directly into the blood from eggs or milk products. It is transported around the body in the form of lipoproteins.

There are three (3) forms of cholesterol, high-density lipoproteins (HDL), low-density lipoproteins (LDL) and very low-density lipoproteins (VLDL). It has been scientifically shown that a high blood cholesterol level increases the risk of developing coronary heart disease. The risk of developing a heart disease is increased if most cholesterol is in the form of low-density lipoproteins or very low-density lipoproteins.

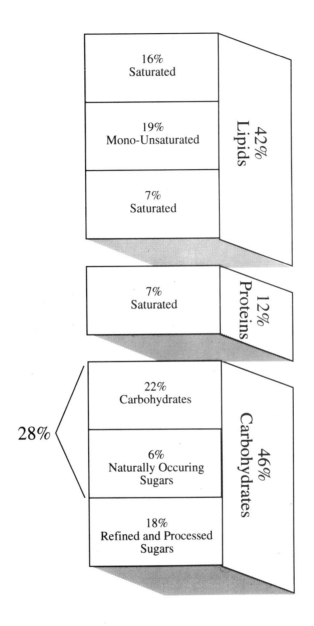

16%
Saturated

19%
Mono-Unsaturated

7%
Saturated

42%
Lipids

7%
Saturated

12%
Proteins

22%
Carbohydrates

6%
Naturally Occuring
Sugars

18%
Refined and Processed
Sugars

46%
Carbohydrates

28%

Figure 1. Lipid, Protein and Carbohydrate components for balancing a typical diet with no alcohol.

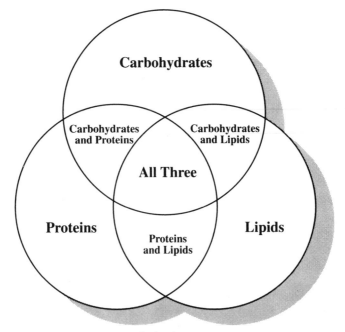

Carbohydrates:
carrots   oranges
sugar   apples

**Carbohydrates
and Proteins:**
dry beans
whole grain bread
macaroni
oatmeal
potatoes

All Three:

chocolate cookies
crackers
vanilla ice cream
whole milk
peanut butter

**Carbohydrates
and Lipids:**
apple pie
mayonnaise
salad dressing

Proteins only:
soy
tofu

Proteins and Lipids:
cheddar cheese
eggs
hamburgers
all-meat hot dogs
beef roasts
tuna fish

Lipids Only:
margarine
oils

Figure 2. How some common foods can be classified as
carbohydrates and/or lipids and/or proteins.

2B. Micronutrients.

Micronutrients are "vitamins" and "minerals". They have virtually no "caloric" or "energy" value, however they are required for energy production. They are absolutely necessary for optimal health, including proper growth and maintenance of cells and tissues. With only a few exceptions, "essential" micronutrients are not manufactured in the human body. They must be obtained from food or food supplements. Vitamins and minerals sometimes fulfill hormone-like functions and aid in the protection of cell membranes. Many vitamins in food can be destroyed in a number of ways, one of which is during cooking.

Vitamins. Vitamins are complex organic molecules that are absolutely "essential" for life and the normal functioning of the body. "Natural" vitamins are found in plants and animals. There are thirteen (13) "essential" vitamins. They are: Vitamins A, B1, B2, B3, B5, B6, B12, C, D, E, H, K, and folic acid.

The "fat-soluble" vitamins are A, D, E, and K. They are absorbed with fats from the small intestines into the blood and then mainly stored in the liver with a small percentage stored in the fatty tissues. The body can store these vitamins for months, depending on the individual's demand for the vitamins. An individual should be cautious with regard to taking too many fat-soluble supplements. If an individual has any concerns about taking fat-soluble supplements, they should seek the advice of a physician who is qualified in dealing with dietary supplements.

The "water-soluble" vitamins are B1, B2, B3, B5, B6, B12, C, H and folic acid. These vitamins are stored in the body for a short period of time. Normally they stay in the body four (4) to six (6) hours. If the body does not utilize the vitamins, most are excreted in the urine. The exception is vitamin B12 that is stored in the liver. A deficiency in the "water-soluble" vitamins is more likely to occur than with "fat-soluble" vitamins. The "water-soluble" vitamins should be taken daily. These vitamins tend to be destroyed by cooking, preserving and processing foods.

Vitamins work with a variety of enzymes. Enzymes consist of a protein molecule and a coenzyme. The coenzyme may be a vitamin, or it could be a substance that contains a vitamin or manufactured from a vitamin. Enzymes are primarily responsible for the oxidation process within the body. Oxidation occurs when oxygen enters the blood and reacts with elements in the blood, such as carbon and hydrogen to generate energy. The byproducts from this reaction are carbon dioxide and water. For example, we breathe in oxygen and exhale carbon dioxide. Water vapor is the byproduct from this reaction. The body is a chemical burning oven that generates energy for mental and physical functions.

There has been extensive research completed to determine the requirements of vitamins and minerals for an individual. The nutritional requirements for every individual vary extensively. It depends on a host of conditions, some of which are age, sex, general health, weight, physical activity, living environment, eating habits, smoking, drinking, pregnancy and many other factors. An individual's diet may provide many of the necessary vitamins. It may then be necessary to offset those deficiencies in the body by taking vitamin and mineral supplements. It could possibly takes weeks, even months, for an individual to see results from supplementing the diet with vitamins and minerals. Any changes in the body chemistry through supplementing the diet with vitamins and minerals would occur on the cellular level. A well balanced diet with proper vitamin and mineral intake is necessary for maintaining good health.

Minerals. Minerals, which by themselves are inorganic, are nutrients that can be found in organic and inorganic substances. There are fifteen (15) minerals that are essential for maintaining good mental and physical health. There are more than forty (40) minerals in our bodies, most of which are in extremely minute amounts.

There are two (2) categories of minerals: "**Major**" and "**Trace**" minerals. The **Major Minerals**, which make up a little more than 0.01% of an individuals body weight are; calcium, chloride, magnesium, phosphorus, potassium and sodium. **Trace Minerals** make up much less than 0.01% of an individual's body weight. They are chromium, copper, fluoride, iodine, iron, manganese, molybdenum, selenium and zinc. Minerals are found in varying quantities in all tissues and internal fluids, such as bones, teeth, muscles, blood and nerve cells. These minerals perform structural and catalytic roles, such as activation of enzymes and hormone production. They are very important in strengthening bones and teeth. Minerals participate in muscle contraction and nerve transmission and provide stimulus to the brain and muscles. They compose approximately 4% to 5% of an individual's body weight. A major percentage of these minerals are found in the skeletal structure. Unlike vitamins, minerals are not destroyed during cooking. They remain after plant and animal tissue is burned.

Minerals work together with many vitamins. For example, iron absorption is aided by vitamin C; phosphorus aids the absorption of the B-complex; calcium absorption is aided by vitamin D and zinc helps vitamin A be released from the liver. Minerals help maintain the body's water balance and assist other nutrients in entering the blood stream. They also aid in creating antibodies and help maintain the acid/alkaline balance in the blood and tissues. As one can see, minerals have many functions in the body.

Minerals are supplied to the body only through an individual's diet. A few good sources of minerals are: milk, cheese, beef, fish, chicken, turkey, ham, a variety of fruits and fruit juices, vegetables, bran and water. Minerals interact with each other and with vitamins. No one (1) mineral can function without effecting other minerals.

Absorption of minerals is dependent on the body's need for that mineral. It is also dependent on what other substances are in the stomach and small intestines at the time they are ingested. Physical and emotional stress also influences the absorption of minerals. It is essential that an individual ingests enough minerals, as well as maintains a balance of each mineral, for the body to function properly. A very important fact is that all minerals may be toxic if too much is ingested. It should also be noted that illness may result if there is a deficiency of one (1) or more minerals, or if there is an over abundance of a mineral.

Iron and calcium are the most common mineral supplements. Iron supplements may be used to treat iron-deficiency anemia and is often needed by pregnant women during breast-feeding. Calcium is the most abundant mineral in the body. The best sources of calcium are milk, dairy products, eggs, fish, and vegetables, fruit and calcium supplements. A deficiency of calcium in the blood is known as hypocalcemia. This blood disorder is relatively rare because most individuals consume foods that contain sufficient calcium. Those individuals who have a very calcium deficient diet have a potential of developing hypocalcemia. In severe cases of calcium deficiency, it causes tetany, which causes cramps in the hands, feet and face. Too much calcium in the blood is extremely rare. It is called hypercalcemia and is often due to cancer that has spread to the bones.

Magnesium deficiency may occur as a result of alcohol abuse, kidney disorders or the prolonged treatment with diuretic drugs. Most other types of mineral deficiencies are extremely rare. Mineral supplements are a common source of a variety of minerals and should be taken only if there is a deficiency of minerals in an individual's diet. If an individual has any concerns about supplementing their diet with minerals, he or she should seek the advice of a qualified doctor and /or a nutritionist.

2C. Essential and Nonessential Nutrients.

There are two (2) types of **nutrients: "Essential"** and **"Nonessential"**.

"Essential" nutrients are absolutely necessary to sustain human life. These nutrients cannot be manufactured by the body they must be consumed in the diet and/or through food supplements. **"Essential"** nutrients include water; carbohydrates; three (3) essential fatty acids; proteins, of which there are eight (8) essential amino acids; at least thirteen (13) essential vitamins and at least fifteen (15) essential minerals. Oxygen, although not typically considered a **"nutrient"**, is absolutely necessary and essential to sustain life. It functions in the same manner as other nutrients at the cellular level.

"Nonessential" nutrients are manufactured in our bodies and are synthesized from **"essential"** nutrients. **"Nonessential"** nutrients include: choline, inositol, carnitine, taurine, lipoic acid, niacin, PABA, and bioflavonoids.

2D. Absorption, Transportation and Metabolism.

Absorption, Transportation and Metabolism of Nutrients.

Absorption. Absorption is the process by which all nutrients, such as, glucose, amino acids, fatty acids, vitamins and minerals enter the bloodstream from the digestive tract. Virtually all of the absorption of nutrients occurs in the small intestines, where complex molecules are broken down into absorbable constituents. Alcohol is absorbed in the stomach while virtually all other ingredients are absorbed in the small intestines.

Nutrients enter the bloodstream through the capillaries in the small intestines. Fat-soluble vitamins enter the blood and move into the cells and tissues. The fat-soluble vitamins that are not immediately utilized in the cells are stored in the liver. The liver changes many of the nutrients into a host of different enzymes. These enzymes are utilized for a variety of purposes throughout the body.

There are numerous factors that influence the intestinal absorption of nutrients. Some of these factors are: 1.) The permeability of the membrane; 2.) The surface tension of the membrane; 3.) The internal temperature; 4.) The various forces of the properties of the intestinal mucosa; 5.) The concentration and the diffusibility of the mixture of ingredients in the small intestines; 6.) The electrical gradient that exists between the ingredients in the small intestines and 7.) The intestinal wall influences the absorption of nutrients.

Carbohydrates are absorbed into the bloodstream in the form of glucose, galactose and fructose. The liver converts galactose and fructose into glucose that is fuel for the body. Fat or lipid digestion produces water-soluble triglyceride products that are easily absorbed in the bloodstream and used for energy. Other fatty acids which are less water-soluble combine with various bile salts to enter the bloodstream. Amino acids are rapidly absorbed from the small intestines directly into the bloodstream. Vitamins and minerals are generally absorbed at specific sites along the small intestine.

Transportation. The nutrients travel through the bloodstream to the cells and tissues, and then to the liver. Some of the nutrients must be actively transported or pumped across membranes because of their structure and the existence of a concentration gradient. This concentration gradient exists between the blood, cellular wall and the tissues. The process of the transfer is called an **"osmotic exchange"**, which occurs when an ingredient moves from an area of high concentration to an area of lower concentration by the use of some other force. Oxygen and nutrients follow a similar path when moving from the blood into the cells. Oxygen, however, is absorbed through the capillaries in the lungs not in the small intestines.

Metabolism. The chemical transformation that occurs with the nutrients in the cells is known as **"the metabolic process"**. The nutrients, while in the cells, are chemically transformed through this processes. The metabolic process consists of oxidation, reduction, interconversion, transformation, energy release, synthesis and storage. This process occurs from the time the nutrients enter the cells and are transformed into active ingredients. These ingredients supply the body with building materials and energy. The waste materials are then discarded from the body.

There are two (2) phases of metabolism that will occur simultaneously, **"anabolic"** and **"catabolic"**. The **"anabolic"** process is where the nutrients undergo chemical changes in which a complex substance is built-up from simpler substances to create the building materials for the blood and tissues. This process usually occurs with the consumption of energy. An example of this is the synthesis of complex proteins from amino acids.

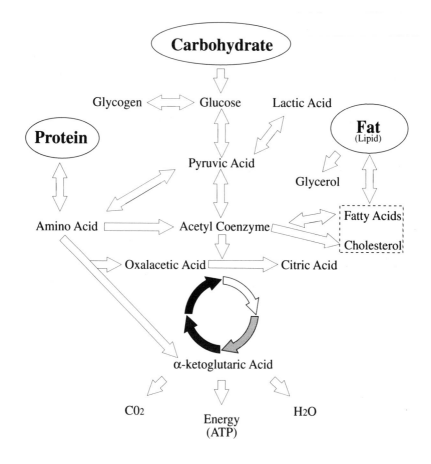

Figure 3 Simplified metabolic pathways of the macronutrients

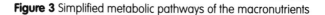

The Vitamin, Mineral and Herb Guide

The "catabolic" process is the chemical reaction where a variety of complex substances are broken down into simpler substances to supply the body with the necessary energy. There is usually a release of energy in the process. This energy is created during the utilization of glucose and the creation of the by-products, water and carbon dioxide. During the metabolic process of essential fatty acids and amino acids, energy is also created. The by-products are carried from the cells by the blood and then out of the body.

The "metabolic rate", known as the "basal metabolic rate (BMR)", is the measure of the energy necessary to maintain the basic body functions at rest. Some of these functions are breathing, heart beat, body temperature and the chemical transformation of the nutrients. There are many factors that influence the BMR, some of which are physical exercise, mental stress, fear and illness. The endocrine hormones and the thyroid hormones mainly control the BMR. These hormones influence the rate at which the chemical changes occur in the cells.

Cellular metabolism is dependent on nutrient availability, enzymatic action and hormone secretion rates. Macronutrients are mutually dependent on the presence and activity of vitamins and the correct concentrations of the electrolytes and other minerals.

2E. The Cell and Cell Membrane.

The "cell" is the basic structural component of the body. The body consists of billions of cells. There are a number of variations in cells and cell types. Most human cells are, however, similar in structure. The red blood cells are highly specialized. These cells are responsible for transporting oxygen throughout the body. The white blood cells are responsible for destroying foreign microorganisms.

The nerve cells are responsible for transmitting nerve impulses that are electrochemical messages in the body. The nerve cells cannot be replaced once they have been destroyed.

Each cell contains a fluid, called "cytoplasm" and an outer membrane. The cytoplasm contains the nucleus of the cell (except in red blood cells) and other elements called organelles.

The "cell membrane", which holds the cell together, consists of a fatty material and proteins in two (2) layers. The key function of the cell membrane is to regulate the passage of various nutrients, including vitamins and minerals, and oxygen into the cell. It also regulates waste materials and other products out of the cell. Small molecules pass freely through the membrane, however larger molecules require a special transport system to cross.

The "**nucleus**" is the control center of the cell and regulates the amounts and types of proteins made in the cell. There are two (2) main functions of proteins. The large structural proteins, such as muscle fibers are the building materials of the body. The small proteins are the enzymes, which regulate all functions and activities of the cell.

In the nucleus of the cell are the "**chromosomes**", known as "**DNA**" or "**deoxyribonucleic acids**" and "**RNA**" or "**ribonucleic acid**". The DNA contains the building codes for protein synthesis and controls the cell's activities by regulating the synthesis of enzymes. DNA consists of two (2) single intertwined chains of RNA. The RNA helps to transport, translate and implement the instructions from the DNA and is often labeled a "**messenger**". There are other constituents in the nucleus called "**organelles**". Each plays a specific role in the body.

3. Vitamins.

Vitamins. Vitamins are organic substances that are necessary for life. They are necessary for growth, vitality and general feeling of well being. All natural vitamins are organic food substances found only in living things - plants and animals. They are normally distinguished as being "**water-soluble**" or "**fat-soluble**". With very few exceptions, the body cannot synthesize vitamins. Vitamins must be supplied in the diet or through dietary supplements. Vitamins function with chemicals called enzymes.

Enzymes are made up of two (2) parts, protein molecules and coenzymes. The coenzyme is often a vitamin, or contains a vitamin, or may be a molecule that has been manufactured from a vitamin. Enzymes are responsible for the oxidation process within the body. They are also a major factor in the biochemical process, such as growth, metabolism, cellular reproduction and digestion. Most enzymes remain in the cell and are utilized within the cell. As the enzyme levels in the cell lowers, the cell efficiency will slowly decrease. This is why the body usually takes many weeks or even many months to show signs of vitamin deficiencies.

A great deal of work has been done to determine the minimum requirements for vitamins and minerals for various age groups and for both sexes. Various physical activity levels, environmental conditions and other circumstances require additional vitamin and mineral demands in the body. The Recommended Daily Allowance (RDA) for vitamins and minerals is based on the standards established by the Food and Nutrition Board of the National Research Council. The desired intake levels for vitamins and minerals are based upon available scientific knowledge and are considered to be adequate to meet the known nutritional needs of most healthy people. These levels are intended to apply to individuals whose physical activity is considered "**light**" and who live in temperate climates. They provide a small safety margin for each vitamin and mineral above the minimum level that will maintain health. Supplements may be ingested to offset any deficiencies where there is any doubt that the requirements for certain vitamins and minerals are not being met through diet alone.

Vitamin and mineral therapy does not produce results over a short period of time. The regeneration or alteration in body chemistry necessary for repair takes weeks or perhaps months before the full benefits are felt. It may also be necessary to change food intake habits. Most vitamins and minerals that are taken in excess of the finite amount utilized in the metabolic processes will be either excreted in the urine or stored in the body. Excessive ingestion of some nutrients may result in toxicity. Risks associated with ingestion of excessive quantities of vitamins and minerals are mentioned at appropriate points in this book.

4. Minerals.

Minerals. Minerals are nutrients that exist in the body and in organic food combinations. There are approximately fifteen (15) minerals that are "**essential**" in human nutrition and are vital to overall mental and physical well being. Minerals are constituents of the bones, teeth, soft tissue, muscle, blood and nerve cells. They are important cofactors in maintaining physiological processes, strengthening skeletal structures and preserving the vigor of the heart, brain, muscle and nerve system. Minerals, like vitamins, act as catalysts for many biological reactions within the human body, including muscle response, the transmission of messages through the nervous system, digestion and metabolism or utilization of nutrients in foods. They are also very important in the production of hormones. Minerals coexist with vitamins and their work is interrelated. Minerals can also be part of the vitamins.

Minerals help to maintain the delicate water balance essential to the proper functioning of mental and physical processes. They help keep blood and tissue fluids from becoming either too acid or too alkaline and permit other nutrients to pass into the bloodstream. Minerals also help draw chemical substances in and out of the cells and aid in the creation of antibodies. All of the minerals known to be needed by the human body must be supplied in the diet; they cannot be manufactured in the body.

5. Who Should Take Vitamins and Minerals?

Who should take vitamins and minerals? Vitamins occur in all organic material. Therefore one could say, if you eat the **"right"** foods in a well-balanced diet, you could potentially get all the vitamins and minerals you would need to stay healthy. Unfortunately, very few individuals are able to arrange and consume this **"mythical diet"**

Most foods that are processed have been depleted of many, if not most, of the vitamins and minerals. Manufacturers attempt to replace those vitamins and minerals to the levels before processing. Many of the techniques for this enrichment are not very effective in properly replacing those vitamins and minerals.

Minerals are as important as vitamins, because without minerals, vitamins can do virtually nothing for you. Vitamins cannot function nor be assimilated without minerals. The body can synthesize some vitamins, however it cannot manufacture any minerals. These minerals have to be ingested in the form of food or supplements. Therefore, unless an individual consumes the **"right"** foods, it may be advantageous to supplement their diet with vitamins and minerals.

Most vitamins are extracted from basic natural sources, such as plants, fruits and vegetables. Vitamins and minerals come in a variety of forms and strengths because everyone's needs are different. The most common is the tablet form. They are easy to store, convenient and normally have a longer shelf life than powders and liquids. Capsules are convenient and easy to store, as well. Vitamins A, D and E are normally found in capsule or softgel form. Caplets are capsule shape tablets and normally "enteric coated" so they dissolve in the intestines, not the stomach. Softgels are soft gelatin capsules and are usually easier to swallow. Powders have advantages of extra potency and the added benefit of no fillers, binders or additives. Liquids are available for easy mixing with beverages and for people unable to swallow capsules or tablets. Another form of providing vitamins and minerals is through the use of nasal inhalers. Also, patches and implants are available and can supply continuous, measured amounts of vitamins and minerals to the body.

A very important step in vitamin manufacturing has been the introduction of **"Time-Release"** supplements. Time or **"Sustained"** Release is a process by which vitamins are encapsulated in micropellets and then combined into a special base for their release in a pattern that assures six (6) to twelve (12) hour absorption time. Most vitamins are water-soluble and cannot be stored by the body. Without time-release, they are quickly absorbed into the bloodstream and are excreted in the urine within two (2) to four (4) hours.

6. Storage of Vitamins, Minerals and Herbs.

Storage of Vitamins, Minerals and Herbs.

Vitamins, minerals and herbs should be stored in a cool, dark place away from direct sunlight and in a tightly closed opaque container. To guard against excessive moisture, place a few grains of rice in the bottom of the container. Vitamins, minerals and herbs can normally last for two (2) to three (3) years in a well sealed, dry opaque container. Once a bottle is opened, one can expect approximately twelve (12) month of shelf life. To insure freshness, always look for the expiration date on the labels of vitamins, minerals and herbs.

The human body tends to excrete water-soluble vitamins in the urine, approximately four (4) to six (6) hours after ingestion. On an empty stomach, vitamins B and C could leave the body in approximately two (2) hours. Fat-soluble vitamins, A, D, E and K (which are stored in the liver) could remain in the body for twenty-four (24) hours or even weeks depending on the individuals demand for that vitamin.

7. How and When to Take Vitamins, Minerals and Herbs.

How and when to take vitamins, minerals and herbs.

As we are all aware, the body works twenty-four (24) hours a day. The body is in need of continuous oxygen and nutrients (vitamins and minerals). Therefore, for the best results, vitamin, mineral and herb intake should be evenly spaced throughout the day. Mineral absorption is potentially increased if taken in the evening hours.

For the best absorption, vitamins, minerals and herbs should be taken after meals with a full glass of water or juice. **"Water-soluble"** vitamins that are excreted fairly rapidly in the urine should be taken after each meal to provide the body with the maximum benefits. For example, the B vitamins and vitamin C are excreted from the body in approximately four (4) hours. You should take the vitamin mineral and herb supplements after the largest meal of the day for maximum absorption potential.

Keep in mind, minerals are essential for proper vitamin absorption. If you are unsure of your body's vitamin and mineral requirements, consult with a physician or a nutritionist who has experience dealing with vitamin and mineral supplemental programs. Also, consult a qualified herbalist to be certain you are taking the proper herbs for your system.

8. Vitamins, Minerals and Herbs.

VITAMINS:

• Vitamin A	-	Retinol
• Vitamin B	-	B-Complex
• Vitamin B1	-	Thiamine
• Vitamin B2	-	Riboflavin
• Vitamin B3	-	Niacin
• Vitamin B5	-	Pantothenic Acid
• Vitamin B6	-	Pyridoxine
• Vitamin B12	-	Cobalamin
• Vitamin H	-	Biotin
• Folic Acid	-	Folacin
• Vitamin C	-	Ascorbic Acid
• Vitamin D	-	Calciferol
• Vitamin E	-	Tocopherol
• Vitamin K	-	Menadione

MINERALS:

- Calcium
- Chlorine
- Chromium
- Copper
- Fluorine
- Iodine
- Iron

- Magnesium
- Manganese
- Molybdenum
- Phosphorus
- Potassium
- Selenium
- Sodium
- Zinc

HERBS:

• Aloe	-	Aloe vera
• Bilberry	-	Vaccinium myrtillus
• Cinnamon	-	Cinnamomum zeylanicum
• Dong Quai	-	Angelica sinensis
• Echinacea	-	Echinacea angustifolia
• Feverfew	-	Tanacetum parthenium
• Garlic	-	Allium sativum
• Ginger	-	Zingiber officinalis
• Ginkgo Biloba	-	Maidenhair tree
• Ginseng	-	Panax ginseng
• Goldenseal	-	Hydrastis canadensis
• Licorice	-	Glycyrrhiza glabra
• Milk Thistle	-	Silybum marianum
• Rosehips	-	Rosa canina
• Saw Palmetto	-	Serenoa repens
• ST. John's Wort	-	Hypericum perforatum
• Valerian	-	Valeriana officinalis

WATER:

- The Source of Life

Vitamin A - Retinol

Description of Vitamin A:

Vitamin A, or Retinaol is a fat-soluble nutrient that occurs in nature in two (2) forms. (1) Performed Vitamin A, which is found only in certain foods and animal origin, and (2) Provitamin A, known as carotene. Carotene is a substance that must be converted into vitamin A before it can be utilized by the body. Beta-carotene is the preferred source of vitamin A because it has less toxicity potential. Only between 1/4 to 1/2 of the carotene is converted to vitamin A. Strenuous physical activity, within four (4) hours of consumption, mineral oil intake, consumption of alcohol, excess iron intake and the use of cortisone and other drugs will interfere with vitamin A absorption. Approximately 90% of the body's vitamin A is stored in the liver. Zinc is required to aid in metabolizing vitamin A out of its storage depots. Most of the absorption of vitamin A occurs in small intestines.

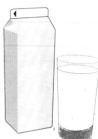

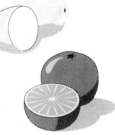

Benefits of Vitamin A:

- *Vitamin A aids in the growth and repair of body tissues and helps maintain smooth, soft, disease-free skin.*

- *It counteracts night blindness, weak eyesight and aids in the treatment of several eye disorders (permits formation of visual purple in the eye).*

- *Vitamin A may help protect the mucous membranes of the mouth, nose, throat and lungs, thereby reducing the susceptibility to infection.*

- *It prompts the secretion of gastric juices necessary for proper digestion of proteins.*

- *Vitamin A is essential for normal growth and reproduction, strong bones, healthy skin, hair, tooth development and healthy gums.*

- *RNA (ribonucleic acid) production is greatly enhanced by vitamin A. RNA is a nucleic acid that transmits instructions to each cell of the body on how to perform so that life, health, and proper function can be maintained.*

- *Vitamin A analogs show promise in the prevention and treatment of certain cancers and in the treatment of certain skin disorders.*

Dosage and Toxicity:

The Recommended Dietary Allowance (RDA) for vitamin A for children is 1500 to 4000 International Units (IU) and 4000 to 10,000 IU for adults. These amounts increase during disease, trauma, pregnancy and lactation. Requirements vary for people who smoke, live in polluted areas, or who easily absorb vitamin A. More than 50,000 IU daily for adults and more than 18,500 IU daily for children, if taken for several months could produce toxic effects. One (1) massive dose or large doses taken over an extended period of time can cause nausea, vomiting, diarrhea, dry and flaky skin, blurred vision, rashes, joint pain, muscle soreness, hair loss, irregular menses, fatigue, headaches, and liver and spleen enlargement. Pregnant women should avoid large doses of vitamin A.

A few good sources of vitamin A are: Eggs, whole milk and milk products, dark green vegetables, yellow fruits and vegetables and liver.

If toxicity is detected, the symptoms will disappear in a few days if the vitamin is no longer ingested. Vitamin C can help prevent the harmful effects of vitamin A toxicity.

Vitamin B - Complex

Description of Vitamin B-Complex:

The B-complex vitamins are water-soluble vitamins. They are not stored in the body; they must be continually replenished. Most B-complex vitamins contain vitamin B1 (thiamine), B2 (riboflavin), B3 (niacin), B5 (pantothenic acid), B6 (pyridoxine), B12 (cyanocobalamin), B15 (pangamic acid), biotin, choline, folic acid, inositol and PABA (para-aminobenzoic acid). There are several reasons for combining the B vitamins into a complex. One reason is their ability to function together during absorption. Several B vitamins are more difficult to absorb into the system and require assistance from other substances. There is also a functional relationship with other B vitamins which enhances the benefits of those vitamins. The B-complex vitamins are necessary for maintaining a healthy nervous system and good muscle tone. The B-complex vitamins are absorbed in the small intestines and carried by the circulatory system to the liver, kidneys and heart, where they combine with specific proteins to become active enzymes. These enzymes break down carbohydrates into simple sugars to provide the body with energy.

Benefits of Vitamin B-Complex:

- *Vitamin B-complex aids in maintaining healthy nerves and nervous system.*

- *It may help reduce mental stress.*

- *Helps to maintain strong muscle tone in the stomach, intestines and heart.*

- *Vitamin B complex is necessary for consistent growth and good appetite in children.*

- *It helps improve the assimilation and digestion of starches, sugars and alcohol.*

- *Vitamin B complex is necessary for maintaining healthy skin and hair.*

- *It may help prevent accumulation of fatty deposits in the artery walls.*

- *Vitamin B complex may increase energy levels through proper utilization of food.*

Dosage and Toxicity:

The B-complex vitamins are a combination of most of the B vitamins. The B vitamins should be taken at the same time and in specific proportionate amounts. Consumption of an excess amount of one (1) B vitamin may have no health benefit and may cause a deficiency in another B vitamin. Individuals who consume excessive amounts of carbohydrates or alcohol require more B vitamins. Alcohol destroys the B vitamins. Alcohol, by it's chemistry, is composed of carbohydrates and contains no vitamins or minerals. This makes it more difficult for the body to use the carbohydrates found in alcohol for energy. The caffeine in coffee has also been shown to destroy some B vitamins. During mental stress and when an infections exists the requirements for additional B vitamins increases. The National Research Council has recommended a certain amount of each B vitamin, refer to the individual B vitamins on the next few pages.

A few good sources of the vitamin B-complex are: Whole grains, meats, fish and poultry, egg yolks, whole milk and milk products, brewers yeast, molasses, nuts and beer.

There are no known toxic effects with B vitamins, mainly because they are not stored, to any degree, in the body.

Vitamin B1 - Thiamine

Description of Vitamin B1:

Vitamin B1, or Thiamine is a water-soluble vitamin that acts as a biological catalyst or coenzyme participating in the complex process of glucose conversion into energy. In this capacity it has a role in metabolic pathways and temperature regulation. It is also involved in the synthesis of fats, in protein metabolism and is needed for normal functioning of the nervous system. Thiamine is rapidly absorbed in the small intestines. It is carried by the circulatory system to the liver, kidneys and heart, where it combines with specific proteins to become active enzymes. These enzymes break down carbohydrates into simple sugars. Thiamine is not stored in the body in any great quantity and therefore must be supplied daily. Smoking and drinking excessive alcohol may result in thiamine depletion.

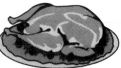
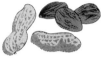
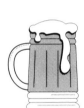

Benefits of Vitamin B1:

- *Vitamin B1 is known as the "morale vitamin" because of its relation to a healthy nervous system and its beneficial effect on mental attitude.*

- *It is necessary for consistent growth in children.*

- *Vitamin B1 helps improve muscle tone in the stomach, intestines and heart.*

- *It may improves food assimilation and digestion of starches, sugars and alcohol.*

- *Vitamin Bl may help prevent undue accumulation of fatty deposits in the artery walls.*

- *It may help in fighting air and seasickness.*

- *Vitamin B1 is useful in relieving dental postoperative pain.*

Dosage and Toxicity:

Individual thiamine needs are determined by body weight, the quantity of the vitamin synthesized in the intestinal tract and daily calorie intake. The higher the calorie intake the higher the proportion of thiamine ingested. The National Research Council recommends 0.5 + milligram of thiamine per 1000 calories daily for all ages. Older individuals tend to use thiamine less efficiently and therefore a higher intake would be necessary. The need for additional thiamine increases during severe diarrhea, fever, stress and surgery. This vitamin works best with B3, B6, vitamin C and niacin. Thiamine can be found in B-complex vitamins.

A few good sources of vitamin B1 are: Whole grains, brewer's yeast, brown rice, meats, fish and poultry, egg yolks, molasses and nuts.

There are no known toxic effects with thiamine because it is not stored, to any degree, in the body.

Vitamin B2 - Riboflavin

Description of Vitamin B2:

Vitamin B2, or Riboflavin is a water-soluble vitamin occurring naturally in those foods in which other B vitamins exist. Riboflavin functions as part of a group of enzymes that are involved in the breakdown and utilization of carbohydrates, fats and proteins. Riboflavin is necessary for cell respiration because it works with enzymes in the utilization of cell oxygen. The amount of riboflavin found in most foods is extremely low, therefore it would be difficult to obtain a sufficient supply without supplementing the diet. Like other B vitamins, it is not stored and must be replaced regularly through whole foods or supplements. Riboflavin is easily absorbed through the walls of the small intestine and is carried by the circulatory system to the tissue of the body. The amount excreted depends upon the intake and relative need of the tissues.

Benefits of Vitamin B2:

- *Vitamin B2 is necessary for the maintenance of healthy skin, nails and hair.*

- *It may help benefit vision and helps alleviate eye fatigue.*

- *It functions with other substances to metabolize carbohydrates, fats and proteins.*

- *Vitamin B2 aids in growth and reproduction.*

- *It may help reduce stress of surgery or mental stress.*

- *Vitamin B2 helps to eliminate sore mouth, lips and tongue.*

Dosage and Toxicity:

The daily riboflavin requirements are related to body size, metabolic rate and rate of growth. These factors are directly related to the protein and caloric intake of the individual. The Recommended Daily Allowance (RDA) for riboflavin is 0.6+ milligrams for every 1,000 calories for adults. Pregnancy and lactation requires additional amounts of riboflavin. Eating red meat and consuming dietary products also requires additional amounts of riboflavin. This vitamin works best with vitamin B6, vitamin C and niacin. Riboflavin is found in B-complex vitamins.

A few good sources of vitamin B2 are: Whole grains, nuts, egg yolks, brewer's yeast, molasses, and organ meats.

There are no known toxic effects with riboflavin because it is not stored, to any degree, in the body.

Vitamin B3 - Niacin

Description of Vitamin B3:

Vitamin B3, or Niacin
(nicotinic acid,
niacinamide,
nicotinamide) is a
member of the vitamin B-
complex and is water-
soluble. It is more stable
than thiamine or riboflavin.
Niacin, as a coenzyme, assists
enzymes in the breakdown and
utilization of proteins, fats and
carbohydrates. Niacin is present
in very small amounts in most
common foods. Niacin is
absorbed in the small intestines
and is stored primarily in the
liver. Any excess is normally
eliminated through the urine. Excessive consumption of
sugar and starches will deplete the body's supply of niacin.
Taking antibiotics will also deplete the available niacin in
the body.

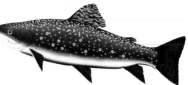

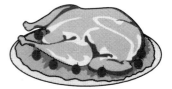

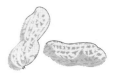

Benefits of Vitamin B3:

- *Vitamin B3 is effective in improving circulation, reducing the cholesterol level in the blood and aids in reducing high blood pressure.*

- *It is vital to the proper activity of the nervous system and brain functions.*

- *It is essential for synthesis of sex hormones (estrogen, progesterone and testosterone).*

- *Vitamin B3 is necessary for the formation and maintenance of healthy skin, tongue and the tissue in the digestive system.*

- *It may help prevent and ease severity of migraine headaches.*

- *Vitamin B3 helps ease some attacks of diarrhea.*

- *It may increase energy levels through proper utilization of food.*

Dosage and Toxicity:

The daily allowance of niacin is based on caloric intake. The Recommended Daily Allowance (RDA) for niacin is approximately 6.6 milligrams per 1000 calories for adults. Increasing caloric intake, pregnancy, lactation, illness, tissue trauma, growth periods and physical exercise require additional niacin.

A few good sources of vitamin B3 are: Poultry and fish, lean meats, peanuts, whole milk and milk products and rice bran.

No real toxic effects are known about niacin. It may cause passing side effects such as: tingling and itching sensations, intense flushing of the skin and throbbing in the head due to a dilation of the blood vessels. This is not considered dangerous and will disappear in approximately 15 minutes.

Vitamin B5
Pantothenic Acid

Description of Vitamin B5:

Vitamin B5, or Pantothenic acid, is part of the vitamin B-complex. Pantothenic acid is water-soluble and is very easily destroyed. It occurs in all living cells and is synthesized in the body by the bacterial flora of the intestines. Most absorption occurs in the small intestines. Pantothenic acid stimulates the adrenal glands and increases production of cortisone and other adrenal hormones important for healthy skin and nerves. Pantothenic acid is a coenzyme and plays a vital role in cellular metabolism. It participates in the release of energy from carbohydrates, fats and proteins. Pantothenic acid also participates in the utilization of other vitamins, especially riboflavin. It is an essential constituent of coenzyme A, which forms active acetate and acts as an activating agent in cellular metabolism. It is essential for the synthesis of cholesterol, steroids (fat-soluble organic compounds) and fatty acids. Pantothenic acid is the liquid part of the lymph in the plasma. It is excreted daily in the urine.

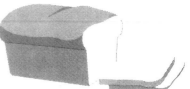
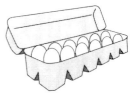
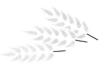
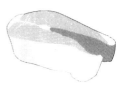

Benefits of Vitamin B5:

- *Vitamin B5 is important in maintaining a healthy digestive tract.*

- *It may improve the body's ability to withstand stressful conditions.*

- *Vitamin B5 helps reduce the toxic effects of antibiotics.*

- *It aids in the prevention of premature aging and wrinkles.*

- *Vitamin B5 helps protect against cellular damage caused by excessive radiation.*

Dosage and Toxicity:

Individual needs for pantothenic acid vary according to periods of stress, daily food intake, age and urinary excretion levels. The Recommended Daily Allowance (RDA) is between 5 and 15 milligrams for adults. A more-than-normal amount of pantothenic acid may be needed after injury, severe illness or antibiotic therapy.

A few good sources of vitamin B5 are: Whole grains, wheat germ, salmon, egg yolks, organ meats and brewer's yeast.

There are no known toxic effects of pantothenic acid.

Vitamin B6 - Pyridoxine

Description of Vitamin B6:

Vitamin B6, or Pyridoxine, part of the vitamin B-complex, is water-soluble. The vitamin B6 consists of three (3) related compounds, pyridoxine, pyridoxal and pyridoxamine. It is required in the proper absorption of vitamin B12 and the production of hydrochloric acid, which aids in the digestion of foods. Most absorption occurs in the small intestines. Pyridoxine is a coenzyme and plays a key role in the breakdown and utilization of carbohydrates, fats and proteins. It must be present for the production of antibodies and red blood cells. Pyridoxine facilitates the release of glycogen for energy from the liver and muscles. It is necessary for the synthesis and proper action of DNA and RNA. Pyridoxine helps maintain the balance of sodium and potassium, which regulates body fluids and promotes the normal functioning of the nervous system and musculoskeletal system. It must be supplied daily because it is excreted in the urine within eight (8) hours after ingestion. Pyridoxine is not stored in the liver.

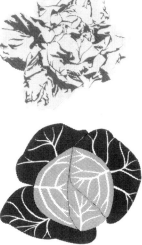

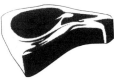

Benefits of Vitamin B6:

* *Vitamin B6 helps the body to properly assimilate carbohydrates, fats and proteins.*

* *It may help prevent various nervous and skin disorders*

* *It aids in the conversion of tryptophan, an essential amino acid, to niacin.*

* *Vitamin B6 may help to promote proper synthesis of nucleic acids.*

* *It may aid in reducing night muscle spasms, leg cramps and hand numbness.*

* *Vitamin B6 helps in the manufacture of antibodies, hemoglobin and hormones.*

Dosage and Toxicity:

The Recommended Daily Allowance (RDA) for vitamin B6 (pyridoxine) is approximately 2 milligrams for adults. The need for pyridoxine increases during pregnancy, lactation, and exposure to radiation, cardiac failure, aging and the use of oral contraceptives. Fasting and reducing diets can deplete the body's supply of vitamin B6. It is most effective when taken with other B vitamins, vitamin C and magnesium.

A few good sources of vitamin B6 are: Meats, whole grains, wheat germ, brewer's yeast, molasses, organ meats and green leafy vegetables.

Over an extended period of time, very high doses of pyridoxine is not recommended. It is involved in the production of hydrochloric acid. Individuals with stomach ulcers should seek the advice of a doctor. Anyone under levodopa treatment for Parkinson's disease should seek the advice of a doctor before taking vitamin B6 (pyridoxine).

Vitamin B12 - Cobalamin

Description of Vitamin B12:

Vitamin B12 or
Cobalamin/Cyanocobalamin
(known as the **"red vitamin"**), part
of the vitamin B-complex, is water-
soluble. Vitamin B12 contains
cobalt, phosphorus and nitrogen. It
is the only vitamin that contains
essential mineral elements. Vitamin B12
is the only naturally occurring organic
compound that contains cobalt. It
cannot be made synthetically but must
be grown. Vitamin B12 is
necessary for normal
metabolism of nerve tissue and
is involved in carbohydrate, fat
and protein metabolism. It is
closely related to the actions of
four (4) amino acids,
pantothenic acid and vitamin C. It will
also help iron function better in the body
and aids folic acid in the synthesis of
choline. Vitamin B12 aids in the
placement of vitamin A into body tissues
by facilitating carotene absorption of
vitamin A conversion. It also aids in the
production of DNA and RNA. It needs
to be combined with calcium during
absorption to be beneficial. Most
absorption occurs in the small
intestines. Vitamin B12 is bound to
serum protein (globulin) and is
transported in the bloodstream to various tissues, liver,
kidneys, heart, brain, pancreas, and bone marrow.

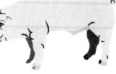

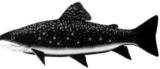
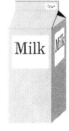
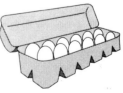

Benefits of Vitamin B12:

- *Vitamin B12 helps form and regenerate red blood cells, which helps to prevent anemia.*

- *It may help in maintaining a healthy nervous system.*

- *Vitamin B12 aids in metabolizing carbohydrates, fats and proteins.*

- *It may help to promote growth and increase appetite in children.*

- *Vitamin B12 may improve concentration, memory and balance.*

- *It helps maintain normal bone marrow*

Dosage and Toxicity:

The Recommended Daily Allowance (RDA) for vitamin B12 (cobalamin) is approximately three (3) micrograms for adults and four (4) micrograms for pregnant and lactating women. Children require one (1) to three (3) micrograms of vitamin B12 daily. Absorption appears to decrease with age and with iron, calcium and B6 deficiencies. The use of laxatives depletes the storage of vitamin B12.

A few good sources of vitamin B12 are: Organ meats, fish and pork, eggs, cheese, whole milk and milk products.

No cases of vitamin B12 toxicity have been reported, even at megadose regiments.

Vitamin H - Biotin

Description of Biotin:

Vitamin H, or Biotin is a water-soluble B-complex vitamin. Biotin is a coenzyme and assists in the synthesis and the oxidation of fatty acids and in carbohydrate metabolism. Without biotin, the body's fat production is impaired. Biotin also aids in the utilization of protein, folic acids, panothenic acid, ascorbic acid and vitamin B12. It plays a role in converting amino acids from protein into blood sugar. Biotin is synthesized in the intestinal bacteria. Some of the biotin is absorbed in the small intestines, but most of the vitamin is excreted in the urine. Biotin is stored, mainly in the liver, kidneys, brain, and adrenal glands.

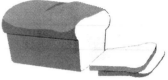

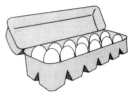

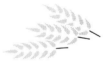

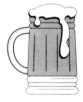

Benefits of Biotin:

- *Biotin may aid in keeping hair from turning gray.*

- *It may help in the preventive treatment for baldness.*

- *It assists in easing muscular pains.*

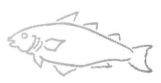

- *Biotin may help promote healthy skin.*

- *It helps improve energy and helps prevent sleeplessness.*

- *Biotin may improve the body's ability to withstand physically stressful conditions.*

Dosage and Toxicity:

The Recommended Daily Allowance (RDA) for biotin is approximately 150 to 300 micrograms for adults. Additional amounts of biotin are required during pregnancy and lactation. Biotin works synergistically and more effectively with vitamins B2, B6, niacin and vitamin A.

A few good sources of biotin (vitamin H) are: Egg yolks, liver, whole grains, rice, brewer's yeast, liver and sardines.

There are no known toxic effects of biotin.

Folic Acid - Folacin

Description of Folic Acid:

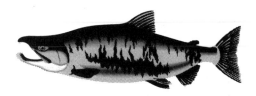

Folic acid, also known as Folacin, Folate and Vitamin M, is part of the water-soluble B complex vitamin. Folic acid is a coenzyme and works together with vitamin B12 and vitamin C in the breakdown and utilization of proteins. Folic acid performs its basic role as a carbon carrier in the formation of heme, the iron-containing protein found in hemoglobin, which is necessary for red blood cell formation.   It is also required for the formation of nucleic acid, which is essential for growth and reproduction of all body cells. Folic acid is necessary for proper brain function and is essential for mental and emotional health. It is concentrated in the spinal and extracellular fluids. Folic acid is absorbed in the gastrointestinal tract by active transport and diffusion. It is stored primarily in the liver.

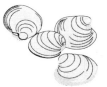

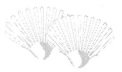

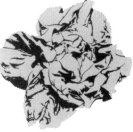

Benefits of Folic Acid:

- *Folic acid increases the appetite and stimulates the production of hydrochloric acid, which helps prevent intestinal parasites and food poisoning.*

- *It aids in the performance of the liver and helps prevent of anemia.*

- *Folic acid helps promote healthy looking skin.*

- *It may delay hair graying when used in conjunction with Pantothenic acid (B5) and PABA.*

- *Folic acid aids in improving individuals learning capacity and helps reduce stress.*

- *It may assist in acting as an analgesic for pain.*

Dosage and Toxicity:

The Recommended Daily Allowance (RDA) of folic acid is approximately 400 micrograms for adults, 800 micrograms during pregnancy and 600 micrograms during lactation. Requirements can vary with individual metabolic rate. The following will increase the body's need for folic acid: Stress, disease, Hemolytic anemia, hyperthyroidism and consumption of alcohol. Folic acid is easily destroyed by high temperature, exposure to light and being left at room temperature for long periods of time.

A few good sources of folic acid are: Whole grains, dark green leafy vegetables, brewer's yeast, oysters, salmon and whole milk.

There is no known toxicity for folic acid, although an excessive intake of folic acid can mask a vitamin B12 deficiency.

Vitamin C - Ascorbic Acid

Description of Vitamin C:

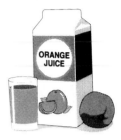

Vitamin C, or Ascorbic acid is a water-soluble nutrient. It is the least stable of vitamins and is very sensitive to oxygen. Its potency can be lost through exposure to light, heat and air. The primary function of vitamin C is maintaining collagen, a protein necessary for the formation of connective tissue in skin, ligaments and bones. It aids in the metabolism of amino acids, in particular phenylalanine and tyrosine. Vitamin C converts the inactive form of folic acid to the active form. It protects thiamine, riboflavin, folic acid, pantothenic acid and vitamins A and E against oxidation. Vitamin C is found in relatively large concentrations in the adrenal glands, and is essential in the formation of adrenaline. In stressful situations, the level of adrenal ascorbic acid is rapidly used up. Vitamin C greatly increases the absorption of iron in the intestinal tract. Vitamin C reaches a maximum level in the blood in 2 to 3 hours. It decreases as it is eliminated in the urine and through perspiration. Vitamin C should be taken throughout the day in smaller quantities to maintain adequate levels. It is absorbed through the mucous membranes in the mouth, stomach and upper part of the small intestines.

Benefits of Vitamin C:

- *It accelerates healing of wounds & burns by forming connective tissue in the scar.*

- *Vitamin C aids in forming red blood cells and preventing hemorrhaging.*

- *It may aid in reducing the effects of some allergy-producing substances.*

- *Vitamin C may aid in the treatment and prevention of the common cold.*

- *Vitamin C increases the absorption of inorganic iron.*

- *It aids in preventing many types of viral and bacterial infections.*

- *It may help counteract the formation of nitrosamines, which may cause cancer.*

- *Vitamin C increases the effectiveness of drugs used to treat urinary tract infections.*

- *It assists in lowering the incidence of blood clots in veins.*

- *It may protect the brain & spinal cord from destruction by free radicals as antioxidant.*

Dosage and Toxicity:

The Recommended Daily Allowance (RDA) is 60+ milligrams for adults. Because vitamin C is excreted in two (2) the three (3) hours, it is important to maintain a constant high level of vitamin C in the blood, small quantities several times a day are recommended. Individual requirements may vary due to differences in weight, amount of physical activity, rate of metabolism, ailments and age. Stress, such as anxiety, infection, injury, surgery, burns or fatigue increases the body's need for vitamin C. Hypoglycemia, high protein diets, ingestion of pain killers, antibiotics, smoking and alcohol increase the need for vitamin C. The normal human body, when fully saturated, contains approximately 5000 milligrams of vitamin C.

A few good sources of vitamin C are: Citrus fruits, strawberries, broccoli, tomatoes, green peppers cantaloupe acerola cherries and rose hips.

Extremely high doses of vitamin C may cause oxalic acid and uric acid stone formation. Occasionally, very high doses, over 10 grams daily, can cause unpleasant side effects, such as diarrhea, excess urination and skin rashes. If this occurs, reduce the dosage.

Vitamin D - Calciferol

Description of Vitamin D:

Vitamin D, or Calciferol, Viosterol and Ergosterol, is a fat-soluble vitamin. It can be acquired by either ingestion or by exposure to sunlight. It is known as the "**sunshine vitamin**" because the action of the sun's ultraviolet rays activates a form of cholesterol, which is present in the skin, converting it to vitamin D. Ingested vitamin D is absorbed with the fats through the intestinal walls. Vitamin D, from dehydrocholesterol by the sun's radiation, is formed in the skin and absorbed into the circulatory system. After absorption, vitamin D is transported to the liver for storage. A small amount is also found in the skin, brain, spleen and bones. The body can store a sizable amount of vitamin D.

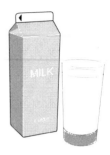

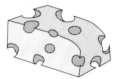

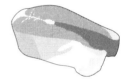

Benefits of Vitamin D:

- *Vitamin D is valuable in maintaining a stable nervous system.*

- *It assists in maintaining normal heart action and normal blood clotting.*

- *Vitamin D aids in the absorption of calcium and the breakdown and assimilation of phosphorus, which is required for bone formation.*

- It is necessary for the normal growth in children, without it bones and teeth do not calcify properly.

- It also may help prevent and reduce cold symptoms when combined with vitamin C.

- Vitamin D assists in the assimilation of vitamin A.

Dosage and Toxicity:

The Recommended Daily Allowance (RDA) for vitamin D is approximately 400 IU for adults. Increase in demand occurs during pregnancy, lactation and physical exercise. Vitamin D works best with vitamin A, vitamin C, choline, calcium and phosphorus. After a suntan is established, vitamin D production through the skin stops.

A few good sources of vitamin D are: Egg yolks, salmon, sardines, herring, organ meats, vitamin D fortified milk and milk products.

Megadoses of vitamin D over an extended period of time can produce toxic effects in adults. Signs of toxicity are unusual thirst, sore eyes, itching skin, nausea, vomiting, diarrhea, urinary urgency, and abnormal calcium deposits in blood-vessel walls, liver, lungs, kidney and stomach. These symptoms will disappear within a few days when the vitamin is no longer ingested.

Vitamin E - Tocopherol

Description of Vitamin E:

Vitamin E, or Tocopherol, is a fat-soluble vitamin. There are eight (8) forms of tocopherols: alpha, beta, delta, epsilon, eta, gamma, theta and zeta. Alpha tocopherols are the most potent form of vitamin E and have the greatest nutritional and biological value. Vitamin E is an antioxidant. An antioxidant opposes the oxidation of substances in the body. Vitamin E prevents saturated fatty acids, vitamin A, vitamin B and vitamin C from breaking down and combining with other substances that may become harmful to the body. When fat oxidizes, it results in the formation of free radicals. These free radicals are very destructive and can cause extensive damage to the body, such as cancer, blood clots, damage to DNA and additional problems. Vitamin E is absorbed through the intestines and into the lymph and carried by the circulatory system to the liver, where it is stored. It can also be absorbed through the skin and mucous membranes.

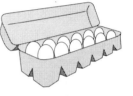

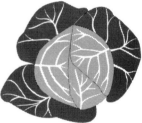

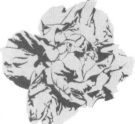

Benefits of Vitamin E:

• *Vitamin E leaves the red blood cells more fully supplied with pure oxygen.*

• *It plays an essential role in cellular respiration of all muscles, i.e. cardiac and skeletal.*

- *Vitamin E, as a diuretic, may help lower an elevated blood pressure.*

- *It aids in protecting the lungs and other tissues from damage by polluted air.*

- *Vitamin E helps promote healing and lessens the formation of scars.*

- *It is a highly effective antithrombin in the bloodstream, inhibiting coagulation of blood by preventing clots from forming.*

- *Vitamin E brings nourishment to the cells, strengthening the capillary walls and protecting the red blood cells from destruction by poisons.*

- *It helps retard the aging of cells by assisting in preventing cellular oxidation.*

- *Vitamin E is necessary for proper focusing of the eyes.*

Dosage and Toxicity:

The Recommended Daily Allowance (RDA) for vitamin E is between 20 and 100+ IU for adults. It is based on the metabolic body size and the level of polyunsaturated fatty acids in the diet. The requirements increase with gains in polyunsaturated fatty acids in the diet. Air pollution increases the need for vitamin E. Initial intake should be small and gradually increase as the body's tolerance level increases. Best taken before meals and/or at bedtime.

A few good sources of vitamin E are: Eggs, wheat germ, molasses, organ meats, olive oil, sweet potatoes and leafy vegetables.

Vitamin E is considered non-toxic except in two (2) conditions: Individuals with high blood pressure or individuals with chronic rheumatic heart disease. These patients should consult their physician prior to taking vitamin E. Toxic symptoms of vitamin E will disappear within a few days after intake is stopped.

Vitamin K - Menadione

Description of Vitamin K:

Vitamin K, or Menadione is a fat-soluble vitamin known as menadione. There are three (3) main K vitamins: K1, K2 and K3. K1 and K2 can be manufactured in the intestinal tract and K3 is produced synthetically. Unsaturated fatty acids and a low-carbohydrate diet increase the amounts of vitamin K produced in the intestinal flora. Vitamin K is involved in glucose phosphorylation, in which phosphate and glucose combine, pass through the cell membranes, and are converted into glucose. It is absorbed in the small intestines and transported by the circulatory system to the liver where it is stored.

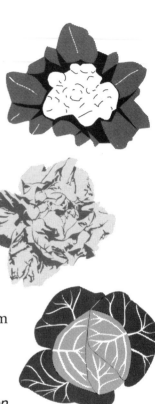

Benefits of Vitamin K:

- *Vitamin K is necessary for the formation of prothrombin, a chemical required in blood clotting.*

- *It is vital for normal liver functioning.*

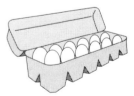

- *Vitamin K is very important for vitality and energy.*

- *It may aid in reducing excessive menstrual flow.*

Dosage and Toxicity:

The Recommended Daily Allowance (RDA) for vitamin K is approximately 300 to 500 milligrams for adults. Therapeutic dosages of vitamin K are often given before and after operations to reduce blood losses.

A few good sources of vitamin K are: Egg yolks, green leafy vegetables, molasses, cauliflower, safflower oils and soybeans.

Toxic manifestations and reactions of vitamin K could occur when megadoses are ingested over an extended period because the supplement will build up in the blood. Toxicity can bring about a form of anemia that results in an increased breakdown in the red blood cells. Flushing, sweating and chest constrictions are symptoms of synthetic vitamin K toxicity. Symptoms will normally disappear within a few days when the megadoses are terminated. Natural vitamin K is stored in the body and produces no toxic signs.

Mineral - Calcium

Description of Calcium:

Calcium is an **"essential mineral"** and is the most abundant mineral in the body. Approximately 99% of the calcium in the body is deposited in the bones and teeth. The remainder, approximately one percent (1%) is involved in the blood-clotting process, in nerve and muscle stimulation, in parathyroid hormone function and in the metabolism of vitamin D. Twenty percent (20%) of an adult's skeleton and thus body calcium is reabsorbed and replaced every year. The ratio of calcium to phosphorus in the bones is 2.5 to 1. Magnesium, phosphorus, and vitamins A, C, D and E must accompany calcium for proper assimilation. The main function of calcium is to act with phosphorus to build and maintain strong bones and teeth. Calcium absorption occurs in the small intestines. The absorption is very inefficient with 20% to 30% of the ingested calcium being absorbed. The remainder is excreted in the urine and feces.

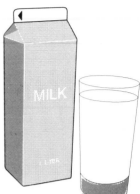

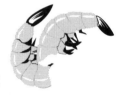

Benefits of Calcium:

- *Calcium helps build and maintain strong bones and healthy teeth.*

- *It is essential for healthy blood and helps regulate the heart when combined with magnesium.*

- *Calcium assists in the process of blood clotting.*

- *It helps prevent the accumulation of too much acid or too much alkali in the blood.*

- *Calcium plays a role in muscle growth, muscle contraction and nerve transmission.*

- *It aids in the body's utilization of iron, activates several enzymes and helps regulate the passage of nutrients in and out of the cell walls.*

Dosage and Toxicity:

The Recommended Daily Allowance (RDA) for calcium is approximately 800 milligrams for adults. The requirements for calcium increase with age, pregnancy and lactation. Many factors interfere with the absorption of calcium, such as phutic and oxalic acid found in plant foods and grains. The lack of exercise, excessive stress, excitement, depression, excessive amount of fat and too rapid a flow of food through the intestines may also interfere with calcium absorption. If the calcium intake is high, the magnesium level must also increase.

A few good sources of calcium are: Milk and milk products, shellfish, molasses, bone meal and green leafy vegetables.

No adverse effects have been observed with a moderate intake of calcium. Ingestion of very large amounts of calcium may lead to hypercalcemia, which is excessive calcification of the bones and some tissues. Overly high intakes may also cause constipation and increase the risk of urinary tract infections.

Mineral - Chloride

Description of Chloride:

Chloride or Chlorine is an **"essential"** mineral, which occurs in the body mainly as sodium chloride and potassium chloride. There is between 450 and 600 milligrams of chloride in every 100 milliliter of blood. It is found in extra-cellular fluids and in gastrointestinal secretions and cerebrospinal fluid. Less than 15% of the body's total chloride content is found in intracellular fluids. Smaller amounts are found in the skin, bone, connective tissue, and muscle and nerve tissue. Chloride helps regulate the correct balance of acid and alkali in the blood. It also helps maintain the pressure that causes fluids to pass in and out of cell membranes until equilibrium is established. Chloride helps stimulate the production of enzymatic fluids in the stomach, gastric hydrochloric acid, for proper digestion of proteins and fibrous foods. It has been found to stimulate the liver to function as a filter for toxic waste products. Chloride is absorbed in the intestines and excreted through urination and perspiration. The controversy still exists over adding chlorine to drinking water supplies. It is a

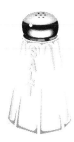
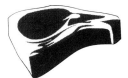
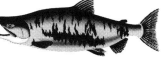
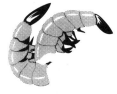
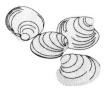

highly reactive chemical and may join with inorganic minerals and other chemicals to form possible harmful substances. It is known that chlorine in drinking water destroys vitamin E and destroys intestinal flora that helps in the digestion of food.

Benefits of Chloride:

- *Chloride aids in cleaning the body of toxic wastes by stimulating the liver functions.*

- *It may help to regulate the blood's alkaline-acid balance.*

- *Chloride assists in stimulating the gastric fluids for better digestion.*

- *It may be helpful in maintaining limber joints and healthy tendons.*

Dosage and Toxicity:

There is no Recommended Dietary Allowance for chloride, mainly because the average individual's salt content is high and usually will provide between 4 and 10 grams daily. A minimum of 750 milligrams for adults has been recommended. Children require between 300 and 750 milligrams of chloride daily, depending on their age.

A few good sources of chloride are: Table salt, seafood, meats, ripe olives and rye flour.

There have been no reported cases of toxicity resulting from an ingestion of too much chloride as it occurs, naturally, in so many foods and in water.

Mineral - Chromium

Description of Chromium:

Chromium is an "**essential**" mineral found in concentrations of twenty (20) parts of chromium per one (1) billion parts of blood. Organic chromium is an active ingredient of GTF (glucose tolerance factor), niacin, and amino acids. Chromium stimulates the activity of

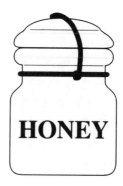

enzymes involved in the metabolism of glucose, and the synthesis of fatty acids and cholesterol. It appears that chromium increases the effectiveness of insulin and its ability to handle glucose. Chromium may aid in preventing hypoglycemia (too much insulin) and diabetes (too little insulin). It competes with iron in the blood. Chromium may be involved in the synthesis of protein through its binding action with RNA molecules. It is also absorbed at different rates in the body. Inorganic chromium is only one percent (1%) or less absorbed in the body. Because of the different forms in which chromium occurs, it is difficult to measure its content in foods. Chromium found in eggs also can not be completely utilized. Approximately three percent (3%) of the ingested chromium is absorbed and retained in the body. It is stored in the spleen, kidneys

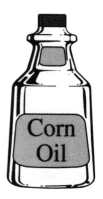

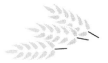

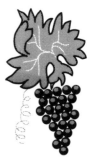

and testes with small amounts in the heart, pancreas, lungs and brain. Chromium has been found in some enzymes and in RNA. Excretion occurs mainly in the urine.

Benefits of Chromium:

- *Chromium works with insulin in metabolizing glucose for energy.*

- *It may help prevent and lower blood pressure.*

- *Chromium may be effective with insulin in preventing hypoglycemia and diabetes.*

- *It also may work with other substances in the body to aid growth.*

Dosage and Toxicity:

To date there is no Recommended Daily Allowance (RDA) for chromium. The daily chromium intake for humans is estimated to range from 80 to 100 micrograms. The amount of chromium stored in the body decreases with age.

A few good sources of chromium are: Honey, grapes, raisins, clams, corn oil, whole grain cereals and brewer's yeast.

There are no known toxic effects with the ingestion of chromium.

Mineral - Copper

Description of Copper:

Copper is a trace mineral found in all body tissues. The body contains between 75 to 100 milligrams (mg.) of copper. Copper acts as a catalyst in the synthesis of hemoglobin and red blood cells by aiding iron absorption. Copper binding to erythrocuprein, a protein known to have superoxide dismutase activity, accomplishes this. It aids in the conversation of the amino acid tyrosine into a dark pigment that colors the hair and skin. Copper also aids in the healing process and in protein metabolism. This mineral works with vitamin C through an oxidation process to form elastin, which is a major component of the elastic muscle fibers throughout the body. Copper is necessary for the production of RNA. It aids in the formation and maintenance of bones. Copper plays an important role in producing energy, by oxidizing cytochrome c in the respiratory chain. Copper is also involved in the synthesis of phospholipids needed to maintain the myelin sheath around the nerve fibers. Approximately 30% of the copper ingested is used by the body and enter the blood stream, about 15 minutes after ingestion. The absorption occurs in the stomach and the upper part of the small intestine. The remainder of the ingested copper is excreted in the feces. Most of the copper is stored in the tissues, with the highest concentration in the kidneys, liver, heart and brain.

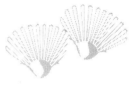

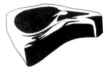

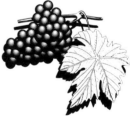

Benefits of Copper:

- *Copper helps maintain energy levels by aiding in effective iron absorption.*

- *It is essential for the utilization of vitamin C.*

- *Copper is necessary for proper bone formation and good maintenance of bones.*

- *It is necessary for the production of RNA.*

Dosage and Toxicity:

The National Research Council recommends between 1.5 and 3 milligrams of copper for adults daily. Children require between 0.7 and 2.0 milligrams, depending on their age. Good sources of copper are: Red meat, whole grain cereals and breads, shellfish, nuts, eggs, poultry and dark green vegetables. Copper is incorporated with iron into hemoglobin.

A few good sources of copper are: Seafood, nuts, molasses, raisins, meats and bone meal.

Wilson Disease is a genetic disorder that results in excessive accumulation of copper in soft tissues and low serum levels. With this disease, too much copper can accumulate in the liver, brain, kidneys and corneas of the eyes. Excessive ingestion of copper may result in serious mental and physical illness. In humans, toxicity results in nausea vomiting, epigastric pain, headache, dizziness, weakness, diarrhea and a characteristic metallic taste. If these symptoms occur, discontinue use immediately and seek the advice of your physician

Mineral - Fluoride

Description of Fluoride:

Fluoride, or Fluorine is an **"essential"** mineral, which is present in nearly every human tissue. It is found mainly in the skeletal structure and in the teeth. The normal blood level of fluoride is 0.28 milligrams per 100 milliliters of blood. Fluoride in the body occurs as fluorides, such as sodium fluorides and calcium fluorides. It has been found that fluoride increases the deposition of calcium, which helps strengthen the bones. It may help reduce acid formation in the mouth caused by certain carbohydrates. Fluoride significantly decreases the incidence of dental carries. There is evidence of reduced osteoporosis in areas that have naturally occurring or added fluorine to the water supply. This added supply of fluoride intake has helped some elderly people to reduce calcium excretion and improved bone density. Fluoride is absorbed mainly in the small intestines, however some may be absorbed in the stomach. Fluoride absorption is very efficient with approximately 90% of the ingested fluoride being found in the blood. Approximately 50% of the absorbed fluoride is found in the teeth and bones. The other 50% is excreted in the urine.

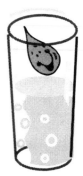
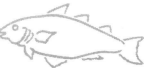
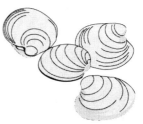
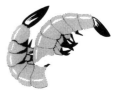

Benefits of Fluoride:

- *Fluoride has been shown to help reduce tooth decay.*

- *It may help strengthen the skeletal structure.*

- *Fluoride has been found to aid in reducing osteoporosis in elderly patients.*

- *It may help in preventing the most common cause of hearing loss in the elderly.*

Dosage and Toxicity:

There is no Recommended Dietary Allowance for fluoride. The average range of fluoride intake is between 1.5 and 4.0 milligrams for adults. For children, the average range is between 0.5 and 4.0 milligrams, depending on their age.

A few good sources of fluoride are: Seafood, tea, fluoridated water and bone meal.

Very high levels of fluoride, from 20 to 80 milligrams daily for several months, may depress growth, cause calcification of the ligaments and tendons. It may also bring about degenerative changes in the kidneys, liver, adrenal glands, heart, central nervous system and the reproductive organs. The amount of fluoride ingested from fluoridated water is approximately 1 milligram per day.

Mineral - Iodine

Description of Iodine:

Iodine is a trace mineral found in all body tissue and is converted into iodide. The body contains between 20 to 50 milligrams (mg.) of iodine. It is found in the muscles (50%), thyroid gland (20%), skin (10%), skeletal structure (7%) and in other endocrine glands (13%). Iodine aids in the development and functioning of the thyroid gland. Iodine is the primary component of the thyroid hormone and is involved in the regulation of cellular oxidation. The thyroid hormone accelerates cellular reactions, increases oxygen consumption and metabolic rate. It is a prime influence in the growth and development of individuals. Iodine can be absorbed through the skin. In the intestinal tract, iodine is converted to iodide and absorbed through the mucosa. Normally the absorption is fast and complete. The iodine that is not absorbed is excreted through the kidneys, with a small amount being lost in sweat, tears and bile.

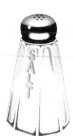

Benefits of Iodine:

- *Iodine is very important in regulating the body's production of energy.*

- *It is a component of the thyroid hormone and aids in stimulating the metabolism.*

- *In the thyroid gland, iodine can aid in burning excess body fat.*

- *It may help in maintaining healthy hair, skin, nails and teeth.*

- *Iodine may assist in maintaining mental alertness and clear speech.*

Dosage and Toxicity:

The National Research Council recommends between 150 and 200 micrograms of iodine daily for adults, the higher dosage is for women who are pregnant or during lactation. Children require between 70 and 120 micrograms, depending on their age. A good source of iodine is iodized salt and water. The iodine content of foods varies greatly and depends on many factors.

A few good sources of iodine are: Seafood, iodized salt and kelp.

There have been no reported cases of toxicity resulting from an ingestion of too much iodine as it occurs naturally in foods and water. However iodine, as a drug or medicine, may have harmful effects which could be serious. Large dosages of iodine given daily, and over a period of time, to individuals with a normal thyroid gland may impair the synthesis of the thyroid hormones.

Mineral - Iron

Description of Iron:

Iron is a an "**essential**" mineral and is concentrated in the blood. It is present in every living cell. All iron in the body is combined with protein. Iron's major function is to combine with protein and copper in making hemoglobin. Hemoglobin is the coloring matter of red blood cells. Hemoglobin transports oxygen in the blood from the lungs to the tissues, which require oxygen to maintain the basic life functions. Iron is also necessary for the formation of myoglobin, which is found only in muscle tissue. Myoglobin is also a transporter of oxygen. It supplies oxygen to the muscle cells for use in the chemical reaction that results in muscle contraction. Iron is present in enzymes that promote protein metabolism. Calcium, copper, cobalt, manganese and vitamin C are necessary to assimilate iron. Ascorbic acid, vitamin C enhances absorption of iron and it is necessary for proper metabolism of vitamin B. The body can utilize either ferric and/or ferrous iron. The evidence indicates that naturally occurring ferrous iron is used more efficiently and that most iron is reduced to ferrous iron before being absorbed. It is absorbed in

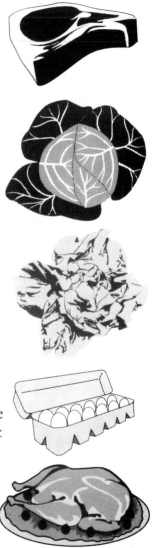

regulated amounts. Approximately ten percent (10%) of iron intake goes into the blood and bone marrow. The absorption occurs in the small intestines and is stored primarily in the liver, spleen, bone marrow and blood.

Benefits of Iron:

- *Iron builds up the quality of the blood and increases resistance to stress and disease.*

- *It works with other nutrients to improve respiratory action.*

- *Iron may help prevent fatigue.*

- *It aids in the cure and prevention of iron-deficiency anemia.*

Dosage and Toxicity:

The Recommended Daily Allowance (RDA) for iron is 18 milligrams for women and 10 milligrams for men. The need for iron increases during menstruation, hemorrhage, periods of rapid growth, or whenever there is a loss of blood. The following interfere with iron absorption: Coffee, tea, lack of hydrochloric acid, the administration of alkali, high intake of cellulose and increased intestinal mobility.

A few good sources of iron are: Eggs, meats, fish and poultry, molasses, cherry juice, dried fruits and green leafy vegetables.

Toxicity of iron is rare in healthy individuals. Excessive doses may be a hazard for children. The toxic level of iron may occur in an individual for some of the following reasons: Due to a genetic error of metabolism, due to blood transfusions, due to a prolonged oral intake of iron, consuming large amounts of red wine that contain iron and those addicted to certain iron tonics.

Mineral - Magnesium

Description of Magnesium:

Magnesium is an **"essential"** mineral that accounts for about 0.05% of the body's total weight. Approximately 70% of the body's supply of magnesium is located in the bones together with calcium and phosphorus. Approximately 30% is found in the soft tissues and body fluids. Magnesium is found mostly in the cell, where it activates enzymes necessary for the metabolism of carbohydrates and amino acids. Magnesium plays an important role in neuromuscular contractions. It may help regulate the acid-alkaline balance in the body. Magnesium aids in the absorption and metabolism of vitamins C, E and the B complex and other minerals, such as calcium, phosphorus, sodium and potassium. Vitamin D is necessary for the proper utilization of magnesium. Nearly 50% of the average daily intake of magnesium is absorbed in the small intestine. The rate of absorption of magnesium is influenced by the parathyroid hormones. The rate of water absorption and the amounts of calcium, phosphate and lactose in the body is also influenced by parathyroid hormones. The adrenal gland secretes a hormone called aldosterone, which helps to regulate the rate of magnesium excretion through the kidneys.

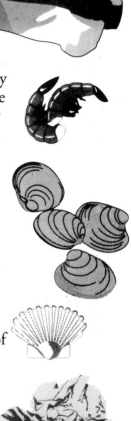

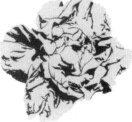

Benefits of Magnesium:

- *Magnesium helps keep teeth and bones healthier.*

- *It is known as the anti-stress mineral and may aid in fighting depression.*

- *Magnesium is necessary for the proper functioning of the nerves and muscles, including the heart.*

- *It is associated with the regulation of body temperature.*

- *Sufficient amounts of magnesium are needed in the conversion of blood sugar to energy.*

Dosage and Toxicity:

The Recommended Daily Allowance (RDA) for magnesium is 350 milligrams for men and 300 milligrams for women. The need for magnesium increases during pregnancy, lactation and extensive physical exercise. Evidence suggests that the balance between calcium and magnesium is especially important. If calcium intake is high, the requirement for magnesium is increased. The need for magnesium is increased when blood cholesterol levels are high, when consumption of protein is high and with high alcohol intake.

A few good sources of magnesium are: Seafood, whole grains, molasses, nuts and dark green vegetables.

Toxicity of magnesium is rare in healthy, normal individuals, but may occur when urinary excretion is unusually decreased and when there is a considerable increase in absorption of the mineral.

Mineral - Manganese

Description of Manganese:

Manganese is a trace mineral. The function of manganese in the body is not very specific because other minerals, such as magnesium, can function in its place. It is understood that manganese plays an important role in activating several enzymes. These enzymes help stimulate the activity and function of vitamin H (biotin), vitamin B1 and vitamin C (ascorbic acid). Manganese acts as a catalyst in the synthesis of cholesterol and fatty acids. It has been shown to aid in stimulating RNA polymerase activity. Manganese is also involved in the formation of collagen, prothrombin and urea. It aids in the digestion of proteins and the synthesis of mucopolysaccharide. It is found in small amounts in the bones, pituitary gland, pancreas, intestinal mucosa, kidneys and liver. The storage of Manganese is limited to approximately 15 milligrams in the body at any particular time. The amount of dietary manganese absorbed in the body is approximately 40% and is absorbed in the small intestines. That which is not absorbed is excreted in the feces.

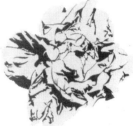

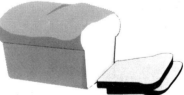

Benefits of Manganese:

- *Manganese is necessary for normal skeletal development.*

- *It may be an important factor in the formation of blood.*

- *Manganese may play an important role in maintaining sex hormone production.*

- *It is essential in the formation of thyroxin, which is a constituent of the thyroid gland.*

- *Manganese may also help nourish the brain and the central nervous system.*

Dosage and Toxicity:

The National Research Council recommends a daily intake of manganese between 2.0 to 5.0 milligrams for adults and 1.0 to 3.0 milligrams for children depending on their age. A higher intake of calcium and phosphorus will increase the need for manganese. However, very high dosages of manganese may reduce the utilization and storage of iron.

A few good sources of manganese are: Green leafy vegetables, spinach, nuts, tea, and pineapples, egg yolks, liver, kidney, and whole grain cereals and bread.

Toxicity of manganese has been shown in industrial workers and miners who inhale large amounts of mineral dust that contains manganese. The symptoms are weakness, irritability, psychological and motor difficulties, leg cramps, headaches, impotency and difficulty in breathing. There have been no reported cases of toxicity resulting from an ingestion of too much manganese as it occurs naturally in food.

Mineral - Molybdenum

Description of Molybdenum:

Molybdenum is a trace mineral that is found in almost all plant and animal tissues. There are approximately 9 milligrams (mg.) of molybdenum in the body. This trace mineral has an essential function in two (2) enzymes systems: xanthine oxidase and aldehyde oxidase. Xanthine oxidase aids in the transformation of iron in the liver from the ferrous to the ferric form and aldehyde oxidase aids in the oxidation process of fats. Both of these enzymes contain FAD (a riboflavin enzyme), which is very important in electron transport. Molybdenum is involved in the metabolism of carbohydrates and fats. It can also interfere with copper absorption because both minerals compete for similar absorption sites in the small intestines. Molybdenum is found in very small amounts in the body. Any excess of molybdenum is excreted in the urine. The storage of molybdenum is in the liver, kidneys and skeletal system.

Benefits of Molybdenum:

- *Molybdenum may have an influence in the prevention of anemia.*

- *Some research has shown evidence that molybdenum may help prevent dental caries.*

- *Molybdenum may aid in decreasing the rate of cancer of the esophagus.*

Dosage and Toxicity:

The National Research Council recommends between 100 and 300 micrograms (mcg.) of molybdenum a day for adults. For children the range is 25 to 150 micrograms depending on their age.

A few good sources of molybdenum are: Liver, kidney, wheat germ, whole grain cereals, whole milk, dried peas and beans and dark-green leafy vegetables.

Toxicity of molybdenum is rare in healthy, normal individuals but can occur with an ingestion of five (5) to ten (10) milligrams (mg.) per day. The toxic effects include, diarrhea, anemia and depressed growth rate. A high intake of molybdenum may cause a deficiency in copper in the body.

Mineral - Phosphorus

Description of Phosphorus:

Phosphorus is an **"essential"** mineral and is the second most abundant mineral in the body and is found in every cell. It often functions more effectively with calcium. A healthy body maintains a specific balance of phosphorus in the bones, 2.5 parts calcium to 1 part phosphorus. However, phosphorus is found in higher ratio in the soft tissues. This balance is necessary for these minerals to function effectively and efficiently in the body. Phosphorus is important in the utilization of carbohydrates, fats and proteins, as well as the production of energy. It stimulates muscle contractions, including the regular contractions of the heart muscle. Niacin and riboflavin cannot be digested unless phosphorus is present. Phosphorus is an essential part of nucleoproteins, which 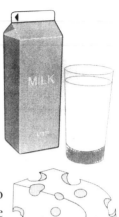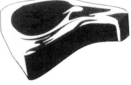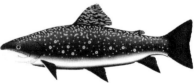 are responsible for cell division and reproduction. It is also responsible for the transference of hereditary traits from parents to offspring. Phosphorus is necessary for proper skeletal growth, tooth development, kidney functioning and transference of nerve impulses. Phospholipids help break up and transport fats and fatty acids. It also helps prevent accumulation of acid or alkali in the blood. Phosphorus will assist in the passage of substances through the cell walls and promotes the secretion of glandular hormones. Approximately 70% of the phosphorus ingested is absorbed through the intestines into the bloodstream. Approximately 88% of the absorbed phosphorus is stored in the bones and teeth. Phosphorus is very dependent on vitamin D and calcium for absorption.

Benefits of Phosphorus:

- *Phosphorus provides energy and vigor by helping in the metabolizing of fats and starches.*

- *It is needed for healthy nerves and efficient mental activity.*

- *Phosphorus may aid in the normal growth of the body and the repair of the body after an injury.*

- *It may help promote healthy gums and teeth.*

Dosage and Toxicity:

The Recommended Daily Allowance (RDA) for phosphorus is 800 milligrams for adults. The need for phosphorus increases during pregnancy and lactation. High fat diets or digestive conditions that prevent the absorption of fat increase the absorption of phosphorus in the intestines.

A few good sources of phosphorus are: Fish, meats and poultry, eggs, whole milk and milk products, nuts, whole grain cereals and bone meal.

There is no known toxicity of phosphorus.

Mineral - Potassium

Description of Potassium:

Potassium is an **"essential"** mineral found mainly in the intracellular fluid. A small amount of potassium is found in the extra-cellular fluid. Potassium constitutes 5% of the total mineral content of the body. Potassium and sodium help regulate water balance within the body. It stimulates nerve impulses for muscle contraction and preserves proper alkalinity of the body fluids. Potassium assists in the conversion of glucose to glycogen, which is the storage form of glucose in the liver. The main functions of potassium are in cell metabolism, enzyme reactions and the synthesis of muscle protein from amino acids in the blood. It stimulates the kidneys to eliminate poisonous body wastes. Potassium works with sodium to help normalize the heartbeat and nourish the muscular system. It unites with phosphorus to send oxygen to the brain, and functions with calcium in the regulation of neuromuscular activity. Potassium is rapidly absorbed in the small intestine. It is excreted mainly through urination and perspiration. The kidneys are able to maintain normal serum levels through their ability to filter, secrete and excrete potassium.

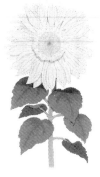

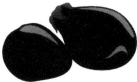

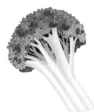

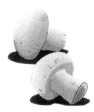

Benefits of Potassium:

- *Potassium is necessary for the normal and healthy growth of the body.*

- *It may aid in keeping the skin healthy and maintaining its elasticity.*

- *Potassium may aid in body repair after an injury.*

- *It may help maintain a clear thinking mind by helping to send oxygen to the brain.*

- *Potassium may assist in reducing a higher than normal blood pressure.*

Dosage and Toxicity:

The Recommended Daily Allowance (RDA) for potassium is between 2000 and 2500 milligrams for adults. Alcohol and coffee increase the urinary output of potassium.Alcohol also depletes the magnesium reserve. Excessive intake of sugar is also antagonistic towards potassium. A low blood sugar level is a stressful condition that strains the adrenal glands causing additional potassium to be lost in the urine while water and salt are held in the tissues.

A few good sources of potassium are: Lean meats, vegetables, whole grains, dried fruits and sunflower seeds.

An intake of 18 grams of potassium in an adult may cause toxicity.

Mineral - Selenium

Description of Selenium:

Selenium is an **"essential"** mineral found in small amounts in all body tissues. Selenium works as an antioxidant and is part of an enzyme called, glutathione, which helps to prevent cellular wall damage. This mineral works together with vitamin E as an antioxidant, which may help prevent or slow down the aging of oxidized tissues. Selenium may help preserve the elasticity of tissues. It has been found to be necessary for the production of prostaglandin, a substance that effects blood pressure. It may help improve energy producing cells by making sure there is adequate oxygen supply. There is some research being done on the anti-cancer properties of Selenium and vitamin E combination. However, a great deal of research is necessary to prove any role in reducing the risk of cancer. The highest concentrations of Selenium are found in the kidneys, liver, spleen pancreas and testicles. The excretion is normally through the urine.

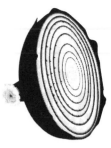
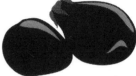
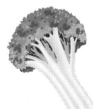
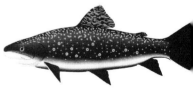

Benefits of Selenium:

- Selenium may aid in keeping youthful elasticity in the tissues.

- It may help improve energy levels and help slow the aging process of tissues.

- Selenium has been found to be necessary for reproduction.

- It works with vitamin E in helping promote normal body growth and fertility.

- Selenium may play an important role in preventing high blood pressure, strokes and hypertensive kidney damage.

Dosage and Toxicity:

The Recommended Daily Allowance (RDA) for selenium is 55 micrograms (mcg.) for women and 70 micrograms for men. For children the range is 20 to 50 micrograms depending on their age.

A few good sources of selenium are: Tuna, herring, fish and shellfish, kidney, liver, meats, wheat germ and bran, whole grains, onions, tomatoes and broccoli.

Toxicity of selenium may occur in healthy, normal individuals. Dosages should not exceed 700 to 1110 micrograms per day over a long period of time, without the advice and supervision of a physician. The toxic symptoms are loss of hair, teeth, nails, dermatitis, lethargy and paralysis. Severe overdoses can produce fever and respiratory problems. If you feel you have any of the above problems due to an overdose of selenium, seek the advice of a physician.

Mineral - Sodium

Description of Sodium:

Sodium is an **"essential"** mineral found in every cell of the body. Sodium is found in the extracellular fluids, the vascular fluids within the blood vessels, arteries, veins and capillaries. It is also found in the intestinal fluids surrounding the cells. Approximately 50% of the body's sodium is found in these fluids with the remainder found in the bones. The body contains approximately 1.8 grams of sodium per kilogram of fat-free body weight. Sodium functions with potassium to equalize the acid-alkali balance in the blood. Sodium, with the aid of potassium, also helps to regulate the water balance in the body, i.e., regulating osmolarity. Sodium, along with potassium, is involved in muscle contraction and expansion. It is an important factor in keeping other minerals soluble, so they will not be deposited on the walls of the blood vessels. There is also evidence of sodium's involvement in nerve stimulation. It helps purge carbon dioxide from the body. Sodium is necessary for the production of hydrochloric acid in the stomach. The absorption of sodium occurs in the small intestine and in the

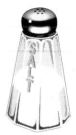

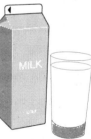

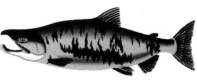

stomach. It is carried by the circulatory system to the kidneys, where it is filtered out and returned to the blood in the levels necessary to maintain certain blood concentrations. Approximately 90% to 95% of the sodium ingested is excreted in the urine.

Benefits of Sodium:

- *Sodium may help nerves and muscles function properly.*

- *It may aid in preventing heat prostration or sunstroke.*

- *Sodium has been shown to aid in the digestive system.*

- *It may help maintain the water balance within the body.*

- *Sodium may help to regulate the blood's alkaline-acid balance.*

Dosage and Toxicity:

There is no established dietary requirement for sodium. Intake is more a function of personal habit, taste and customs than for need. It is estimated that an adult should take approximately 500 milligrams per day and children, between 200 and 500 milligrams per day, depending on their age. Deficiencies are uncommon because most foods contain some sodium.

A few good sources of sodium are: Table salt, seafood, celery, milk products, kelp, baking powder and baking soda.

There is evidence correlating high sodium intake and low calcium intake with elevated blood pressure and edema. The easiest way to reduce sodium intake is to eliminate the use of table salt.

Mineral - Zinc

Description of Zinc:

Zinc is an "**essential**" mineral
occurring in the body in larger
amounts than any other trace
element, except iron. The human
body contains approximately 1.8
grams of zinc. It is related to the
normal absorption and action of
vitamins, especially the B complex.
Zinc is a constituent of at least 200
enzymes involved in digestion and
metabolism, including carbonic
anhydrase, which is necessary for tissue
respiration. Zinc is a component of
insulin and is part of the enzyme that is
needed to break down alcohol. It is also
involved in carbohydrate digestion and
phosphorus metabolism. Zinc is
essential in the synthesis of nucleic acid,
which controls the formation of
different proteins in the cell. It may also
be required in the synthesis of DNA, which is
the master substance of life. DNA carries all
inherited traits and directs the activities of
each cell. The best source of all trace elements,
including zinc, is natural unprocessed foods.
Zinc is readily absorbed in the small
intestines. The body will only absorb
as much zinc as it needs, with the
remainder being unabsorbed. It is
mainly stored in the liver, pancreas,
kidney, bones and voluntary muscles.

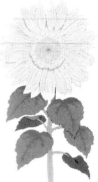
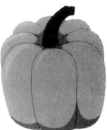

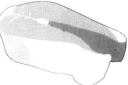

Benefits of Zinc:

- *Zinc has been found to be essential for normal growth and proper development of the reproductive organs.*

- *It may be necessary for normal functioning of the prostate gland and may aid in preventing prostate problems.*

- *Zinc is important in healing internal and external wounds and burns.*

- *It may promote growth and mental alertness.*

- *Zinc may reduce the duration of colds and the flu by as much as one half.*

Dosage and Toxicity:

The Recommended Daily Allowance (RDA) for zinc is between 15 and 60 milligrams (mg.) for adults. Thirty (30) milligrams is recommended during pregnancy and forty-five (45) milligrams during lactation. A high intake of calcium and phytic acid, found in certain grains, may prevent absorption of zinc. Excessive zinc intake can result in iron and copper losses.

A few good sources of zinc are: Seafood, oysters, herring, mushrooms, soybeans, wheat germ, eggs, meats, pumpkin and sunflower seed, and brewer's yeast.

Zinc is virtually non-toxic, however, an intake of 2 grams (gm.) or more can produce toxic effects.

Herbs - Aloe

Description of Aloe:

Physicians and healers, for a variety of ailments, have used Aloe, or Aloe vera for more than 2,500 years. Some of the more prominent topical uses of the gel are to heal wounds and burns, to soothe a sunburn, in treating dry skin problems, especially eczema, and to help fight infection. The aloe plant originated out of the tropical areas in Africa. The Greeks and Romans used the gel from the plant to heal the wounds of soldiers after a 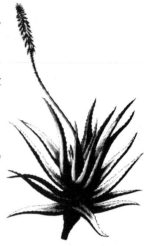 battle. Today, the aloe gel is used in a great variety of cosmetics and skin creams and is known as one of the best natural moisturizers. The healing benefits and the successful treatment of a woman with severe x-ray burns using the aloe gel was first documented by an American medical journal in 1935. Over the past 60 years, scientific evidence has shown that the aloe gel helps in the treatment of certain types of skin infections. It has also been used to treat fungal infections, such as ringworm. The powder from the aloe leaves can be made into a capsule and then into a tonic to be used to treatment anemia, poor digestion and liver disorders. It is used as a purgative and will help promote bile flow. Research is continuing on other potential benefits of aloe. One study shows aloe may kill the fungus, Candida albicans, which causes vaginal yeast infections. Another shows aloe may help reduce blood sugar levels with individuals who have diabetes. And there may be some benefit of aloe in treating leukemia. A great deal of research has to be completed to validate any of these new potential benefits of aloe.

Benefits of Aloe:

- *Aloe helps soothe and promote the healing of sunburns and other minor burns.*

- *It helps make the skin soft, smooth and supple.*

- *Aloe may help heal skin wounds, bug bites and other minor skin irritations.*

- *It has been shown to help prevent infections in skin wounds.*

- *In tonic or capsule form, aloe may be used as a laxative and only in very small dosages.*

- *As a tonic, aloe may increase menstrual flow in small doses.*

Dosage and Toxicity:

The thick aloe gel is an ideal topical first aid cure for burns, wounds and sunburn. The leaves are made into capsules, softgels or a powder (100 to 500 mg per dose). It is used as a purgative, laxative and a digestive aid. The gel, from the leaves, may be applied directly to the skin. The gel can be boiled down to a thick cream and stored for future use. There is no established Recommended Daily Allowance (RDA) for aloe. As aloe stimulates uterine contractions, it should be avoided during pregnancy. It should also be avoided during breast-feeding. Not highly recommended as a laxative.

Herbs - Bilberry

Description of Bilberry:

Bilberry, or Vaccinium myrtillus was once a highly regarded folk remedy used as a urinary antiseptic. It was once touted as a cure-all for such ailments as scurvy, kidney stones, and diabetes. It was even supposed to stop the milk flow in nursing mothers. It is also thought to help people, who suffer from **"night blindness,"** which is a difficulty in seeing in the dark. Bilberry may help accelerate the regeneration of visual purple also known as retinol purple, which is required for good eyesight. In the Elizabethan era, the apothecaries made syrup from the berries and added honey. This mixture was used as a very effective 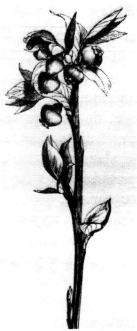 remedy for diarrhea. The berries, of the bilberry plant, contain a pigment, which is believed to kill or inhibit the growth of bacteria. For this reason, the berries were thought to be especially useful in treating dysentery. A large quantity of the berries however, may have a laxative effect. The ripe berries of the plant also contain flavonoids. The most important flavonoid is the anthocyanosides. Studies show that anthocyanosides speed the regeneration of visual purple in the eye, which allows the eye to adjust better and faster to light and dark. Other studies show that anthocyanosides strengthen the capillary walls and also increase the blood flow. The leaves of the bilberry plant are believed to help lower blood sugar levels. The most recent research indicates the leaves may increase insulin production.

Benefits of Bilberry:

- *Bilberry may help preserve eyesight and prevent eye damage.*

- *Bilberry may be helpful for people who suffer from "night blindness".*

- *The leaves may be useful as a urinary antiseptic.*

- *Bilberry leaves may be helpful in reducing blood sugar levels and increasing insulin production.*

- *The fresh berries may be eaten to help reduce constipation.*

- *The unsweetened juice of the berries has been used effectively for diarrhea.*

Dosage and Toxicity:

The fruit and the leaves of bilberry are used. Bilberry can be taken as a "**standard extract**" softgel, as a capsule, as a tea or liquid concentrate. The berries can also be eaten with milk and sugar for constipation. Bilberry can also be made into a lotion by adding an equal amount of witch hazel and the same amount of bilberry juice for treating a sunburn and skin inflammations. There is no established Recommended Daily Allowance (RDA) for bilberry. The leaves of the bilberry plant has been shown to lower blood sugar levels, therefore, those individuals who are insulin-dependent diabetics should not take them without the advice of qualified professional individuals.

Herbs - Cinnamon

Description of Cinnamon:

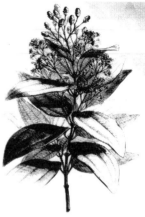

Cinnamon, or Cinnamomum zeylanicum is an ancient Chinese herb and is believed to be first used around 2700 BC to treat fever, menstrual problems, diarrhea, as an anti-septic, uterine stimulant and to relieve nausea and vomiting. The Egyptians used the herb in the embalming process. The Hebrews, Greeks and Romans used the herb to treat indigestion. It has been used as a treatment for colds, the flue and stomach cramps, as well as, other stomach disorders. Cinnamon is also used in the treatment of arthritis and rheumatism. It is most commonly known as a powerful antiseptic. Cinnamon kills disease-causing bacteria, viruses and certain types of fungi. It contains a natural anesthetic oil called eugenol, which may be helpful in relieving a variety of minor pains. There is evidence that cinnamon may help stimulate some digestive enzymes, which helps breakdown fats. It is generally believed that cinnamon causes uterine muscle contractions and helps reduce the bleeding during the menstrual cycle. However, there is a good deal of controversy regarding the effects of cinnamon on the uterus. Some herbalist's suggest it calms the uterus, while others say it stimulates the uterus. Research in ongoing to determine the actual effects. There is also a great deal of research being done on the effects of cinnamon on reducing blood pressure. And there is some evidence that cinnamon may have hypoglycemic properties, which would be beneficial for diabetics.

Benefits of Cinnamon:

- *Cinnamon is helpful in the treatment of colds and the flu.*

- *It is used to reduce the effects of diarrhea.*

- *Cinnamon is a powerful antiseptic, it kills disease-causing bacteria and viruses.*

- *It may be used to treat minor cuts and scrapes on the skin.*

- *Cinnamon is a good digestive aid by breaking down fats in the digestive system.*

- *It may be used topically by soaking it in a pad and placing the pad on joints to help relieve arthritic and rheumatic pain.*

Dosage and Toxicity:

Cinnamon comes in a powder, sticks of the inner bark, as a **"standardized extract"** softgel or as an essential oil,. The essential oil of cinnamon, approximately 5 drops, may be dissolved in boiling water and inhale the steam for relief of coughs and respiratory irritations. Dilute approximately 5 ml in hot water for colds and chills. Dilute approximately 1 ml of cinnamon oil in 25 ml of another herbal oil for massage. There is no established Recommended Daily Allowance (RDA) for cinnamon. Cinnamon should be avoided, in therapeutic doses, during pregnancy, because it may potentially stimulate the uterus.

Herbs - Dong Quai

Description of Dong Quai:

Dong Quai, or Angelica sinensis is a Chinese herb and has been used for more than 2,000 years to treat a vast number of gynecological problems, such as infertility, premenstrual syndrome (PMS), menstrual cramps, menopause and irregular menstrual cycles. Today it is one of the most important herb tonics in China. Dong quai contains two (2) active 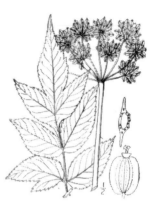 compounds called coumarin and ferulic acid. Coumarin has properties that help prevent blood clotting. It also functions a lot like estrogen, which helps relieve menopausal complaints, such as hot flashes. Ferulic acid is commonly known as a pain reliever and relaxes the muscle. There is also evidence that the ferulic acid in dong quai may help relax the uterine muscle, the heart muscle and may help lower blood pressure. For this reason, dong quai is used as a nourishing blood tonic. Modern herbalist's recommend dong quai to help regulate the menstrual cycle and to soothe other female gynecological complaints, such as menstrual cramps and the discomfort of premenstrual syndrome (PMS). Dong quai may be useful in helping women resume normal menstruation after going off the pill. There are some studies that support dong quai's effectiveness in treating certain allergies and respiratory problems. The root, when used as a general tonic, may help clear the liver of toxins and may relieve constipation. Dong quai contains

vitamins A, B12 and E. It may help prevent anemia.
Dong quai has been used by both men and women to
help prevent insomnia and to treat high blood pressure.
Dong quai has been referred to as the **"female ginseng"**.

Benefits of Dong Quai:

- *Dong quai may help restore menstrual regularity.*

- *It may reduce or eliminate the discomfort of
  premenstrual syndrome (PMS).*

- *Dong quai relieves the symptoms of menopause and
  other menstrual irregularities.*

- *It has been prescribed to help prevent anemia.*

- *Dong quai may help reduce high blood pressure.*

- *It has been shown to relieve constipation, especially
  in the elderly.*

Dosage and Toxicity:

The leaves and the roots of dong quai are used. Dong
quai can be taken as a **"standardized extract"** softgel, as a
capsule, as a tea or liquid concentrate. The leaves can also
be made into a cream by adding approximately ten (10)
drops of the liquid to a cream or herbal oil for skin
irritations and arthritic pain. Dong quai can also be
made into a tincture or oil. There is no established
Recommended Daily Allowance (RDA) for Dong quai.
Avoid regular or large doses during pregnancy, because it
may be a uterine stimulant. Diabetics should consult a
qualified professional herbalist and/or medical doctor
before taking Dong quai because of its sugar content.

Herbs - Echinacea

Description of Echinacea:

Echinacea, or Echinacea angustifolia has its roots in North America. The Native Americans used this herb to heal wounds, snakebites, and insect bites. They also used this herb as a mouthwash for painful teeth and gums and drank an echinacea tea to treat colds, the flu, measles, mumps and smallpox. Since the 1930's this herb has been very popular in Europe and mostly ignored 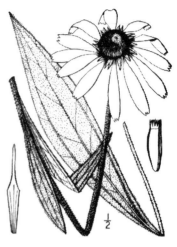 in the United States. Recently, western medicine has acknowledged the positive benefits on the immune system. Studies have shown that echinacea boosts the infection fighting white blood cells and T-cells. Echinacea has been shown to help the body rid itself of microbial infections, particularly bacterial, viral, fungi and protozoa attacks. This herb contains a natural antibiotic (echinacoside), which is comparable to penicillin. It has also demonstrated similarities to the body's own virus fighting chemical, interferon, which boosts the ability of cells in the body to resist infection. Echinacea strengthens the tissues and tissue walls against the bacterial and viral microorganisms. Many European studies, mostly German, have shown Echinacea has remarkable healing properties and has shown to lessen the severity of colds and the flu. It is also effective in treating tonsillitis, bronchitis, tuberculosis, meningitis and ear infections. Echinacea has also been shown to be very effective in treating vaginal yeast infections, when used in conjunction with an anti-yeast cream (echinacea is taken orally). Other European studies have shown echinacea may have an anti-inflammatory effect, which may lay credence for the treatment of arthritis.

Benefits of Echinacea:

- *Echinacea may shorten the duration of colds and the flu.*
- *It has been shown to help reduce the recurrence of vaginal yeast infections.*
- *It may help fight bacterial and viral infections.*
- *Echinacea has been shown to help promote the healing of skin wounds.*
- *Echinacea boosts the immune system.*
- *It may be effective in treating arthritis.*

Dosage and Toxicity:

The flower and the root of echinacea are used. Echinacea can be taken in a "**standardized extract**" softgel as a capsule (200 mg - 3 times a day), as a tea or liquid concentrate. As a tea, take approximately 10 ml in a warm liquid for infections or gargle for sore throats. There is no established Recommended Daily Allowance (RDA) for echinacea.

The medical literature contains no reports of echinacea toxicity. Pregnant and nursing women should consult their physician before taking echinacea.

Herbs - Feverfew

Description of Feverfew:

Feverfew, or Tanacetum parthenium was been used by the ancient Greek herbalist's to treat a number of menstrual problems and birth-related problems. It was also used to treat arthritis. In the 1600's, feverfew was used to strengthen the womb of pregnant women, to expel the placenta after birth and for other uterine disorders. In the 1700's, feverfew was prescribed to relieve many types of head pains, such as migraines. In most of these treatments, feverfew was mainly applied externally because of the 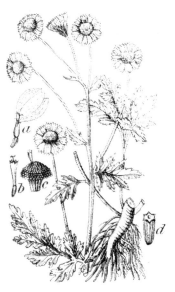 strong bitter taste. It was also thought to be potentially dangerous, if taken internally. The name was originally named parthenion. It was later changed to featherfoil because of its feathery leaves and then to its present name, feverfew. When this name was acquired, it was mistakenly thought to reduce fevers. Research has shown that feverfew may inhibit the release of serotonin from platelets and prostaglandin from the white blood cells. These two (2) substances are believed to contribute to migraine headaches and they may potentially play a role in rheumatoid arthritis. Feverfew has been used as an anti-inflammatory. There is some evidence that feverfew may open or relax blood vessels. Taken internally, in a drink, pill or capsule form, feverfew is used as a digestive stimulant. Some herbalist prescribe feverfew to promote menstruation and as a uterine stimulant.

Benefits of Feverfew:

- Feverfew is helpful in reducing the pain associated headaches.

- It may be helpful in reducing the severity of nausea and vomiting.

- Feverfew may reduce the pain and inflammation of rheumatoid arthritis.

- It has been shown to reduce blood pressure.

- Feverfew is a good digestive aid and stimulant.

- It may be help promote menstruation and as a uterine stimulant.

Dosage and Toxicity:

The leaves of feverfew are used. Feverfew can be taken as a **"standardized extract"** softgel, as a tincture or one may eat the leaves. Approximately 15 g of herb to 500 ml of water can be drunk for menstrual pain and congestion. Take approximately 5 to 10 drops of tincture in water for head pains. Saut'e a few leaves with and a little oil and apply topically to relieve muscle pains. There is no established Recommended Daily Allowance (RDA) for feverfew. Feverfew should be avoided during pregnancy because it may potentially stimulate the uterus. Patients taking blood-thinning drugs should also avoid it because it may affect clotting rates. Mouth ulcers are a potential side effect of eating the fresh leaves. Discontinue use if mouth ulcers occurs.

Herbs - Garlic

Description of Garlic:

Garlic, or Allium sativum has been used for more than 5,000 years to treat an assortment of ailments. The Egyptians fed it to their slaves to keep them healthy. Garlic has been used to treat tuberculosis, reduce blood cholesterol levels, respiratory infections, and in treating cancer and heart disease. Louis Pasteur tested the effects of garlic on bacteria and viruses, and found that it killed those alimentary microorganisms. Dr. Albert Schweitzer used garlic to treat cholera, typhus and amebic dysentery while he was working as a missionary in Africa. Garlic can contribute to the overall effectiveness of other vitamins and minerals through better absorption and utilization in the blood. Studies on animals and humans show that garlic can help modify blood lipids, reduce the risk of developing atherosclerosis and cardiovascular disease. When garlic or essential oils are added to the diet, serum cholesterol and triglycerides can be reduced, while increasing the high-density lipoproteins (HDL's - good cholesterol). Garlic will also lower blood pressure. It has been shown to reduce low-density lipoproteins (LDL's - bad cholesterol) and fibrinogen, as well as, increase the anti-clotting factor which reduces the risk of blood clots. Studies have shown that epidemiological studies support these findings and show an inverse correlation between average garlic consumption and incidence of cardiovascular disease in different geographical studies. Garlic will aid in the development of natural bacterial flora, while it kills pathogenic organisms thereby aiding digestion. The compound in garlic mainly responsible for this effect is called "**cycloalliin**". Garlic has also been shown to be toxic to some forms of cancer.

Benefits of Garlic:

- *Garlic helps lower cholesterol levels (LDL's) in the blood.*

- *Aids in modifying the blood coagulation mechanisms to reduce the risk of blood clots.*

- *Garlic helps to fight a variety of infections, such as, respiratory, colds and flu.*

- *Daily intake of garlic helps lower systolic and diastolic blood pressure.*

- *It may help reduce the risk of developing atherosclerosis and cardiovascular disease.*

- *Garlic may be helpful in treating certain forms of cancers.*

Dosage and Toxicity:

The cloves of the garlic are used. Garlic comes in raw clove form, as a tablet, as a "**standardized extract**" softgel, as a capsule or in powder form. Dosage remains a controversial subject. The apparent absence of side effects makes garlic at moderate to high doses an attractive therapy in the prevention and treatment of cardiovascular disease. There is no established Recommended Daily Allowance (RDA) for garlic.

There are no known toxic effects of garlic. In therapeutic doses, pregnant women or those breast-feeding without the approval and supervision of their physician should not use garlic.

Herbs - Ginger

Description of Ginger:

Ginger, or Zingiber officinale is a very well known remedy for an upset stomach, indigestion and for cramps. It has been used by the Chinese for more than 3,000 years for stomach ailments, to treat arthritis and kidney problems. The Chinese women drank ginger tea to relieve menstrual cramps, morning sickness and a variety of other gynecological problems. The Chinese sailor would chew the 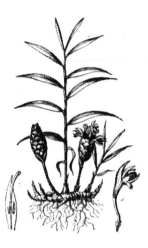 gingerroot to prevent seasickness. The American Indians used ginger in cooking to preserve the food and prevent digestive problems. They would chew the gingerroot to eliminate the smell of garlic and onions from their breath so they would not offend their Gods. Gingerbread originated from the ancient Greeks when they put ginger in bread to alleviate indigestion. The English added ginger to water containing sweeteners and called ginger beer and used as a remedy for nausea, diarrhea and vomiting. Later, the ginger beer was carbonated and called ginger ale. In the early 1900's, it was touted as the cure-all for nausea, diarrhea, indigestion, dysentery, fever, headaches, toothaches and menstrual problems. Today, the herbalist's prescribe ginger to help reduce the effects of colds, the flu, motion or seasickness, as well as, a digestive aid and to help eliminate nausea. There is scientific evidence showing ginger does help prevent seasickness, motion sickness and morning sickness during pregnancy. Some physicians are recommending ginger to chemotherapy patients to help eliminate nausea. Ginger is used as a digestive aid because it helps break down proteins.

Research has further shown that ginger helps kill the influenza virus and some other infectious viruses and bacteria. There are several studies on ginger's anti-inflammatory effects, which would help treat arthritis. The New England Journal of Medicine published a study showing that ginger helps lower blood pressure and may help prevent internal blood clots that are responsible for heart attacks and strokes. Other studies are being done on potential benefits in treating cancer.

Benefits of Ginger:

- *Ginger helps prevent seasickness, motion sickness and dizziness.*

- *It acts as a digestive aid by breaking down proteins.*

- *Ginger helps kill the influenza virus and helps prevent vomiting.*

- *It has been shown to be very effective in treating colds and other infectious diseases.*

- *Ginger has anti-inflammatory properties that may help treat arthritis.*

- *Ginger helps relax peripheral blood vessels and may help reduce cholesterol levels.*

Dosage and Toxicity:

The roots and the rhizome of ginger are used. Ginger can be taken as a "**standardized extract**" softgel, as a capsule, as an essential oil and can be eaten in raw root form. Steam 1 or 2 slices in water for chills. Use 2 to 10 drops of the essential oil in warm water for indigestion and nausea. Take 200 mg to 400 mg in capsule form for motion sickness. Add 5 to 10 drops of the essential oil with 25 ml of another herbal oil for massage. There is no established Recommended Daily Allowance (RDA) for ginger. Individuals with peptic ulcers should avoid excessive amounts of ginger.

Herbs - Ginkgo Biloba

Description of Ginkgo Biloba:

Ginkgo Biloba, or Maidenhair tree has been used by the Chinese for more than five thousand (5,000) years to treat asthma, inflammations due to allergies and swelling of the hands and feet due to damp cold. The Chinese and Japanese ate roasted ginkgo biloba seeds to aid in digestion and to help prevent drunkenness. Much research is being done in Europe, particularly in France, because of the positive effects on the 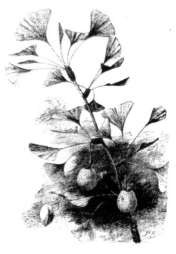 cardiovascular system. The research shows that ginkgo biloba increases the blood flow to the brain and to other organs in the body. Ginkgo biloba has been shown to have tremendous healing potential, particularly for various conditions associated with aging. With the increase in blood flow to the brain, memory improves, as well as, other mental functions. It may also help speed recovery for an individual who has experienced a stroke. Ginkgo biloba improves the blood flow to the heart muscle, which may help prevent a heart attack by reducing the risk of blood clots. Research has also shown ginkgo biloba improves the blood flow to the lower extremities and may help reduce pain, cramping and weakness in the legs. It has been shown to be very effective in treating asthma and other respiratory complaints. A number of other studies have demonstrated ginkgo biloba's effectiveness in the treatment of impotence, deterioration of the retina, chronic ringing in the ears (tinnitus), chronic dizziness (vertigo) and hearing loss due to decreased blood flow to the nerves in the ear. These ailments are aided by increases in the flow of blood to those areas of the body.

Benefits of Ginkgo Biloba:

- *Ginkgo biloba helps improve the blood circulation throughout the body.*

- *It helps improve a variety of mental functions and helps improve memory.*

- *Ginkgo biloba may help retard the aging process.*

- *It may help prevent bronchial constrictions with individuals who suffer from asthma.*

- *Ginkgo biloba may be helpful in reducing hemorrhoids and varicose veins.*

- *It may help prevent chronic ringing in the ears and chronic vertigo.*

Dosage and Toxicity:

The leaves and the seeds of ginkgo biloba are used. Ginkgo biloba can be taken as a **"standardized extract"** softgel, as a capsule, as a tea, use the dried leaves or as a tincture. The seeds are found only on the female plant and, may be eaten or made into a tincture and mixed with other herbs. There is no established Recommended Daily Allowance (RDA) for ginkgo biloba.

In extremely large amount of the seeds, some individuals have experienced irritability, diarrhea, headaches and nausea. Recommended amounts are considered non-toxic.

Herbs - Ginseng

Description of Ginseng:

Ginseng [Panax ("**all-healing**") ginseng] is a known as the "**wonder herb**". It has been used by the Chinese for over 5000 years as a health promoter to treat the elderly for arthritis, senility, loss of sexual interest, impotence and lethargy. Ginseng means the "**root of man**", because the roots resemble the shape of a man. Ginseng was used by the American Indians to combat fatigue, to help 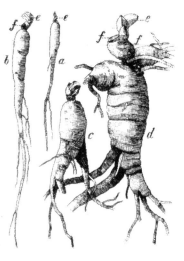 digestion, to increase the appetite and to make a love potion. The chemicals that are responsible for the healing potential of ginseng are called ginsenosides. Research has shown ginseng helps stimulate the immune system by activating the production of interferon and antibodies, which both fight bacterial and viral infections. Ginseng reacts in the system by strengthening and stimulating the endocrine glands that control all basic physiological processes, including the metabolism of minerals and vitamins. It may also be effective in counteracting the deficiency of vitamin B1 and B2. It has been shown to reduce the LDL's - low-density lipoprotein (bad cholesterol) levels and increase the HDL's - high-density lipoprotein (good cholesterol) levels. Ginseng may have an anti-clotting effect in the blood, which would help reduce the possibility of heart attacks. It may strengthen the heart and central nervous system. Ginseng has also been known to build-up a persons general mental and physical vitality and resistance to disease. It is believed that Ginseng may rejuvenate the entire physiological system and increase sexual energies. Current research, by the Chinese and Soviets, is being completed on ginseng's anti-tumor potential.

Benefits of Ginseng:

- *Ginseng may increase an individuals mental endurance, thereby aiding in the acceleration and retention in learning.*

- *It has been known to enhance an individuals physical endurance and energy level.*

- *It may assist in lowering high blood sugar levels and lower LDL cholesterol levels.*

- *Ginseng may have a stimulating effect on the human sex hormones.*

- *It has been found to normalize the level of arterial pressure and can be effective in the treatment of hypotension and hypertension.*

- *Ginseng may be effective in treating colds, coughs, rheumatism, neuralgia, gout, diabetes, anemia, insomnia, stress, headache, backache and double vision.*

Dosage and Toxicity:

The root of ginseng is used. Ginseng can be taken as a **"standardized extract"** in softgel form, as a capsule, as a tea, liquid or a concentrate. Ginseng should be taken daily over a two (2) month period of time, followed by a two (2) week break, to stimulate rejuvenation and virility of the body. There is no established Recommended Daily Allowance (RDA) for ginseng. Ginseng is considered a non-toxic substance that increases the resistance of an organism to a wide variety of stress factors, whether they are physical, chemical or biological. Pregnant women and individuals with hypertension should avoid ginseng in high doses.

Herbs - Goldenseal

Description of Goldenseal:

Goldenseal, or Hydrastis canadensis was used by the Cherokee and Iroquois Indian tribes in the Northeast as a yellow dye and, medicinally, to treat skin wounds, local inflammations and to improve the appetite. It was also used to treat whooping cough, liver disorders, fevers and heart problems. The two (2) active ingredients in goldenseal are berberine and hydrastine. Research has found that berberine kills many bacteria that cause diarrhea and is very effective against the protozoan that cause dysentery.

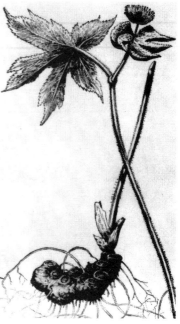

Researchers have also found this ingredient very effective against cholera, streptococcus and chlamydia. Goldenseal has mild anti-inflammatory properties which makes it a good treatment for the throat, stomach, and vaginal area. It has also been considered a gastrointestinal remedy for diarrhea and excessive intestinal activity. Goldenseal has been shown to enhance the immune system by stimulating the white blood cells. Because of the anti-microbial properties, it has shown to be effective in treating the symptoms of colds and the flu. Goldenseal has been used in stopping excessive menstrual flow, however it is also known to stimulate uterine contractions. Pregnant women should not use this herb. Goldenseal may help digest fats by stimulating bile secretions and soothing the intestines. Research on humans and animals has shown goldenseal helps shrink brain tumors and skin cancers. With research on-going in this area, someday goldenseal may be useful in treating cancer.

Benefits of Goldenseal:

- *Goldenseal has anti-inflammatory properties and may soothe irritated mucous membranes.*

- *It may help relieve the symptoms of colds and the flu.*

- *Goldenseal may aid in stopping excessive menstrual blood flow.*

- *It may help reduce menstrual pain or premenstrual syndrome (PMS).*

- *Goldenseal may be helpful in reducing skin inflammations, such as eczema.*

- *It may help aid indigestion and constipation.*

Dosage and Toxicity:

The root and rhizome of goldenseal are used. Goldenseal can be taken as a **"standardized extract"** softgel, as a capsule, as a tea or used as a tincture. The tincture can be diluted (1 to 3 ml) and used a mouthwash, douche or flush for skin irritations and an eye wash. There is no established Recommended Daily Allowance (RDA) for goldenseal.

Goldenseal stimulates the involuntary muscles of the uterus and, therefore, should not be used by pregnant women. Individuals with high blood pressure, heart disease, diabetes, glaucoma or a history of stroke should not use goldenseal. If an individual has any concerns about taking this herb, they should consult with their physician.

Herbs - Licorice

Description of Licorice:

Licorice, or Glycyrrhiza glabra is one of the oldest known herbs used to treat certain ailments. According to legend, the Chinese used this healing herb some 5,000 years ago. It was used to treat a cough, respiratory problems, malaria, liver and uterine problems, and some cancers. Around 300 BC, the Greeks and Romans used the herb to treat colds, sore throat, cough, 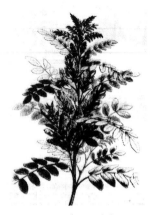 asthma and other repertory and gastrointestinal problems. In the 14th century the Germans and Italians used the herb to treat respiratory, stomach and heart problems. The Native Americans would drink a tea brewed with licorice root to suppress a cough, as a laxative, to treat ear aches and to mask the taste of other healing herbs. The licorice root contains a chemical called glycyrrhetinic acid (GA) which has strong cough-suppressant properties. Today, it is found in a number of cough suppressants formulas. GA may have ulcer healing properties. Large amounts of GA may cause a person to retain water. Water retention is potentially serious because it could lead to elevated blood pressure. GA releases serotonin from platelets and prostaglandin from the white blood cells. These two substances are believed to contribute to migraine headaches and may play a role in rheumatoid arthritis. Scientists have found a method of removing 97% of the GA, while maintaining licorice's healing benefits, which created a new herbal medicine called deglycyrrhizinated licorice (DGL). European researchers have reported very impressive results treating duodenal ulcers with licorice. Licorice also has anti-inflammatory and anti-arthritic properties. It has shown great promise when taken internally and when applied topically to joints. Recent research has demonstrated licorice stimulates the production of interferon, which is the body's anti-viral compound, which may be beneficial in the treatment of the herpes simplex virus. There is also research being done on licorice's ability to fight disease-causing bacteria and fungus. Chinese researchers have shown that licorice may help improve liver functions and help control hepatitis. New research is being done on licorice's anti-tumor properties in laboratory animals. A great deal of research must be done to validate these properties in licorice.

Benefits of Licorice:

- *Licorice is an excellent cough suppressant.*

- *It is used as a treatment to reduce the pain of peptic ulcers.*

- *Licorice has expectorant properties that will breakup congestion due to colds.*

- *It has very good anti-inflammatory and anti-arthritic properties.*

- *Licorice may help reduce the pain and stiffness associated with arthritis.*

- *It has been shown to help reduce blood cholesterol levels.*

Dosage and Toxicity:

The root of the licorice plant is used. Licorice can be taken as a **"standardized extract"** softgel, as a fluid extract or the raw root can be chewed. Use 2 to 5 ml of the extract as a digestive stimulant. There is no established Recommended Daily Allowance (RDA) for licorice. Licorice should be avoided if an individual has high blood pressure, rapid heartbeats or those taking digoxin-based drugs.

Herbs - Milk Thistle

Description of Milk Thistle:

Milk Thistle, or Silyburn marianum has been used for more than 2,000 years by the Roman herbalist's to clean and rejuvenate the liver. In the 18th century the English herbalist's used this herb to treat jaundice and in the early 19th century, the German physicians used this herb to treat individuals with liver disease. The first use of milk thistle, as a healing herb, in the United States was around the end of the 19th century. It was used to treat liver, spleen and kidney disorders. By the turn of the century, the use of milk thistle virtually disappeared from western medicine. In the mid 1960's, German researchers began looking at the properties of milk thistle and it's functions in the liver. The active ingredient in this herb is a flavonoid, called silymarin. Silymarin has been shown to have a direct effect on liver cells by rejuvenating and protecting these cells. The liver produces a substance called bile. This bile breaks down fats in the small intestines. It also will detoxify poisons, such as alcohol, nicotine and other toxic chemicals that enter the blood stream, by breaking those chemicals down into non-toxic substances. The liver is an extremely important organ in the body, not only because of the bile production and its

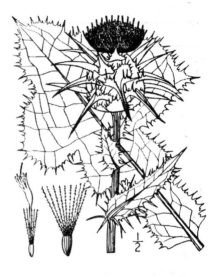

benefits, but also the fat-soluble vitamins A, D, E and K, are stored in the liver. A good deal of research is ongoing in the United States and in Europe to determine the benefits of milk thistle in treating individuals with alcohol related liver disease, viral hepatitis, liver cirrhosis and those individuals in drug therapy.

Benefits of Milk Thistle:

- *Milk thistle may be helpful in rejuvenating liver cells.*

- *It may be helpful in protecting the cells against toxins, such as, alcohol and nicotine.*

- *Milk thistle increases the production of bile, which breaks down fats in the small intestines.*

- *It may be helpful in the treatment of chronic hepatitis.*

- *Milk thistle may also be helpful in the treatment of drug dependency.*

Dosage and Toxicity:

The part seeds of the dried flower of milk thistle are used. Milk thistle can be taken as a **"standardized extract"** softgel, as a capsule, or as an liquid extract. The softgels or capsules come in a "standardized extract" of 70% to 80% of silymarin, which is approximately 420 milligrams of silymarin. There is no established Recommended Daily Allowance (RDA) for milk thistle.

There is no known toxicity or side effects when using milk thistle.

Herbs - Rosehips

Description of Rosehips:

The Rosehip, or Rose canina is the very small bud that is left after the leaves fall of the rose. It is touted as one of the best natural sources of vitamins C. Some researchers may disagree. The Romans used the wild rose to treat bites from a rabid dog. The Greek herbalist's would mix the petals from the rose with oils to treat diseases of the uterus. In India, the ancient physicians would make an oil from the rose petals to treat

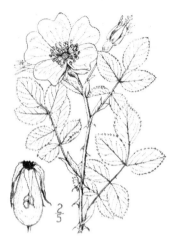

skin wounds and inflammations. They would also mix the rose petals with water and use as a laxative. In the early days of Germany, the herbalist's would make a rosehip tea and would use it for a vast number of ailments. In the 1700's, the English herbalist's used a rosehip tea to prevent vomiting, diarrhea and to stop a cough. In the 1800's, the European herbalist's would use dry rose petal tea to treat headaches, dizziness, cancer sores and menstrual cramps. The Chinese would use rosehip tea to treat urinary dysfunctions and chronic diarrhea. In the early 20th century, roses almost disappeared as a medicinal remedy. Then in the 1930's vitamin C, in potentially appreciable amounts, was discovered in rosehips. The Apothecary's in the 1930"s would recommend a tincture of rosehips for a sore throat. Scientific studies have shown that vitamin C helps relieve the symptoms and reduce the duration of the common cold. The New England Journal of Medicine suggest using 2,000 milligrams per day or more from the onset of the symptoms of a cold until all symptoms are gone. A hot rosehip tea may help relieve a sore throat, nasal congestion and a cough associated with a cold or flu virus. Other potential properties of rosehips are: It may work as an antidepressant, aphrodisiac, sedative, digestive stimulant, expectorant, anti-bacterial, anti-viral, anti-septic, kidney tonic, blood tonic, menstrual regulator and as an anti-inflammatory. Research has not documented many of these supposed actions of rosehips.

Benefits of Rosehips:

- *Rosehips may help relieve the symptoms and decrease the duration of a cold.*

- *It may be helpful as a tea to relieve a sore throat, nasal congestion and a cough.*

- *Rosehip tea may reduce the effects of diarrhea and stomach cramps.*

- *As an essential oil, it may be helpful in reducing anxiety and depression.*

- *The rose petals and rosehips, as a tea, may help relieve digestive problems.*

Dosage and Toxicity:

The petals and the rosehips of the rose are used. An essential oil is made from the petals. Use 2 to 4 milligrams of rosehips in hot water for diarrhea and coughs. Add a few drops of the oil to creams or herbal oils for dry skin and massage. There is no established Recommended Daily Allowance (RDA) for rosehips. Rose oil is non-toxic and may be taken internally. Prior to using the rose oil, consult a professional regarding the dosages and with regard to which species of rose is good for the above listed benefits.

Herbs - Saw Palmetto

Description of Saw Palmetto:

Saw Palmetto, or Serenoa repens, has been used since the turn of the century to tone and strengthen the male reproductive system, as well as, to treat chronic urinary tract infections. Some early herbalist's believed this berry would increase sperm production and increase their sex drive. This herb has also been used extensively in Europe, particularly in Germany, for an over-the-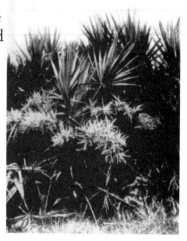
counter treatment for benign prostate enlargement. Saw Palmetto has been prescribed by herbalist to treat **"honeymoon cystitis"**, which is an irritation of the penis due to excessive sexual activity. The active ingredient in saw palmetto is a lipophilic extract, which is the fatty acid portion. There is evidence that an active form of testosterone, called dihydrotestosterone (DHT) is responsible for prostate enlargement. It is believed that saw palmetto can reduce this form of testosterone in the prostate tissue. It has also been shown to reduce the inflammatory effects of an enlarged prostate, as well as, reducing the effects of estrogen and progesterone on the prostate. It may also work as an aphrodisiac, to stimulate the male sex hormone. Some research has shown that saw palmetto has been very effective as a urinary tract antiseptic and in some cases as a diuretic. The berries are normally used as a tonic or taken in a capsule form.

Benefits of Saw Palmetto:

- *Saw Palmetto may help relieve some problems associated with benign prostate enlargement.*

- *It may have an aphrodisiac effect and stimulate the male sex hormone.*

- *Saw Palmetto may be used as a diuretic.*

- *It may helpful in treating urinary tract infections.*

- *Saw Palmetto may help clear the chest of congestion.*

Dosage and Toxicity:

The berries of saw palmetto are used. Saw palmetto can be taken as a "**standardized extract**" softgel (160 mg to 320 mg of extract are used), as a capsule, or as a tea. The berries can be made into a tincture and combined with other herbs. Use 10 g of berries with 500 ml of hot water as a diuretic and antiseptic. There is no established Recommended Daily Allowance (RDA) for saw palmetto.

There is no known toxic effects with individuals using saw palmetto. Men who suffer from an enlarged prostate gland, which is associated with difficulty in urinating, as well as, pain and swelling of the prostate gland, should seek the advice of their physician before taking this herb.

Herbs - ST. John's Wort

Description of ST. John's Wort:

ST. John's wort, or Hypericum perforatum, was named by the early Christians in honor of John the Baptist. It was believed that the red oil, which is released from the plant's leaves when pinched, was the blood of Saint John when he was beheaded on August 29. ST. John's wort has been used as a medicinal herb for more than 2,000 years. The Romans used the herb with wine to treat snakebites. The Greeks used the herb 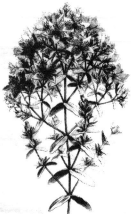 externally to treat burns and internally, as a diuretic, for menstrual cramps and malaria. Both the Greeks and Romans believed this herb would protect them from witches' spells. In the 1600's, the English would soak the leaves in oil and use the mixture to treat skin wounds. The native American Indians used this herb, as a tonic, to treat diarrhea and fevers. They would make an ointment to treat snakebites, wounds and other skin problems. Throughout the 19th century, ST. John's wort was used to treat an number or ailments, such as, skin wounds, snake bites, asthma, diarrhea, hemorrhoids, menstrual cramps, congestion, certain forms of paralysis, as a tranquilizer and to treat insomnia and depression. A great deal of research is being done in the former Soviet Union and in Germany. They found that ST. John's wort may contain anti-viral, anti-bacterial, anti-fungal, anti-inflammatory and anti-depressant properties. Several research studies support the herb's wound healing properties. The red oil contains; hypericin, immune stimulating flavonoids and other antibiotic chemicals. There is also scientific evidence that this herb is a good anti-depressant. The hypericin in the herb interferes with monoamine oxidase (MAO), which is believed to be a key factor in depression. In 1988, researchers at New York University and the Weizmann Institute discovered that the hypericin in the herb, reacts against several viruses, including the human immunodeficiency virus (HIV). A few of the results from individuals taking this herb are, increased immune functions, improved appetite, weight gain and an increase in energy. A good deal of research is now being done to validate these findings and it's potential benefits as an AIDS treatment.

Benefits of ST. John's Wort:

- *ST. John's wort promotes the healing of skin wounds and bites.*

- *This herb may help the body fight viral infections.*

- *It may be helpful in reducing anxiety, irritability and emotional problems.*

- *ST. Johns wort may be helpful in the treatment of depression.*

- *It has been shown to be a muscle relaxant and used to treat menstrual cramps.*

- *ST. John's wort may be beneficial in the treatment of HIV.*

Dosage and Toxicity:

The flowers and leaves of ST. John's Wort are used. St. John's wort can be taken as a **"standardized extract"** softgel, as an infused oil or use the flowers and leaves. There is no established Recommended Daily Allowance (RDA) for ST. John's wort. Internally, as a tonic, mix 10 to 15 drops with a liquid. For external use, use a few drops mixed with a light herbal oil. This herb may cause dermatitis when taken internally and then exposing the skin to the sun.

Herbs - Valerian

Description of Valerian:

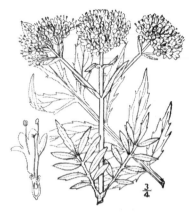

Valerian, or Valeriana officinalis was used by the native Americans to treat skin wounds. In the early 1800's it was listed in the US Pharmacopoeia as a tranquilizing agent. In the 1900's it was prescribed to hypochondriacs and those with epilepsy as a calming agent. Today, in the United States and in Europe, herbalist recommend valerian for nervousness, reducing tension, insomnia, anxiety and headaches. In Germany valerian is the active ingredient in many over-the-counter tranquilizers. Valerian has very few side effects, with the exception that it has a disagreeable smell and considered not very tasteful. The chemical, valepotriates, is the active ingredient in valerian, which depresses the nervous system. This chemical gives valerian it's sedative effect. The root has also been used to strengthen the heart muscle and may help reduce high blood pressure. There is also evidence that valerian may help heal wounds and ulcers. Herbalist's have also used valerian as a topical treatment to soothe muscle cramps. Research on animals has shown valerian may have anti-convulsive effects, which could be used in treating epilepsy.

Benefits of Valerian:

- *Valerian has been used successfully in calming the nerves and as a sedative.*

- *It is used to treat anxiety, reducing tension and insomnia.*

- *Valerian may help strengthen the heart muscle and reduce high blood pressure*

- *It is used to relieve muscle cramps and is applied topically.*

- *Valerian may help and enhance the healing of wounds.*

- *It may also be used as an expectorant and help relieve coughing spells.*

Dosage and Toxicity:

The root and rhizome of valerian are used. Valerian can be taken as a "**standardized extract**" softgel, as a capsule, or as a tea. The valerian roots can be made into a tincture and combined with other herbs. Use 2 to 4 ml of the tincture with hot water for anxiety and insomnia. There is no established Recommended Daily Allowance (RDA) for valerian.

It is recommended that an individual taking this herb for two (2) or three (3) weeks should take a break. High doses over a prolonged period of time may cause headaches, nausea and restlessness. Avoid taking valerian with other medication that is sleep inducing.

Water -
The Source of Life.

Water is the second (2nd) most important element in sustaining life, only oxygen is more essential. Without either water or oxygen, life will cease. Water makes up between 45% and 65% of an adults body. In children and newborn babies the water content is between 59% and 77%. Normally, men have slightly more water in their bodies than women and 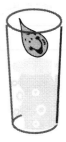 younger people have slightly more water than older people. In the body, blood is 83% water, kidney - 82%, muscles - 75%, brain - 74% and bones - 22%. Overall, approximately 70% of lean body tissue is water. It is the primary constituent in the fluids that surrounds all living cells. Water is extremely important in respiration, metabolism, temperature regulation, the elimination of bodily wastes and digestion. It also lubricates joints and acts like a shock absorber in the eyes and spinal column. Another very important function of water is its ability to dissolve and transport the nutrients, such as oxygen and mineral salts, through the circulatory system. Water also helps in maintaining the osmotic pressure, acidity and the composition of all chemical reactions. The circulation in the blood stream and tissues is perpetual and is always maintained at a proper balance. Humans can live only five (5) to seven (7) days without water, depending on the particular climate of the region. A certain amount of water, approximately one (1) liter per day, is eliminated through perspiration, urination, feces and through evaporation. Some water is removed by the kidneys, through which the blood supply passes and is filtered fifteen (15) times every hour. When the body overheats, approximately two (2) million sweat glands open and perspiration occurs. The heat of the blood evaporates the perspiration, which attempts to cool the body and keep the internal organs at a constant temperature. This perspiration is made up of 99% water. Some water is lost through tearing and breathing. Dry air will evaporate body moisture much faster than moist air.

Hard Water and Soft Water: Hard water contains higher concentrations of calcium and magnesium, therefore it is more alkaline than soft water. Soft Water normally has more sodium concentration and is therefore more acidic than hard water.

Benefits of Water:

- *Water will keep all bodily functions; respiration, digestion, metabolism temperature regulation, waste removal, etc. functioning.*
- *It is necessary for dissolving and transporting nutrients throughout the body.*
- *Water maintains all chemical reactions in the body in equilibrium (hydrolysis and condensation).*
- *It may aid in dieting by depressing the appetite before meals.*

How Much is Good for You:

There is no standard for the amount of water an individual should ingest. Any excess is excreted in the urine. It is very important to pay attention to the body signals. When you thirst for water, indulge yourself, unless you have been instructed not to by your physician. Approximately three (3) liters (or approximately three (3) quarts) is needed per day to replenish the body's water supply under normal conditions. Individuals who have a higher physical activity, live in climates which have higher temperatures and higher humidity or with diets which are high in sodium content may require more water. Foods can also add in replenishing water in the body.

Bibliography and Additional Reading

In the past several years, there has been an increased public awareness and interest in understanding the benefits and uses of vitamins, minerals and herbs. This has prompted a vast number of books in all of these areas. A good deal of research has been done over the past twenty (20) years. In the last five (5) years there has been a tremendous amount of research done to validate the uses, benefits, dosages and the possible toxicity of the various vitamins, minerals and herbs.

Internet Websites:

Individuals who have access to the Internet can retrieve related articles on vitamins, minerals and herbs by using some of the Internet information systems, for example, MEDLINE and NAPRALERT. A few other sources:
www.prev.com/house/index.html,
www.med.harvard.edu/publications/Health_Publications,
www.hotwired.com/drweil/, www.healthy.net, www.herbs.org/herbs/,
www.tufts.edu, www.healthnet@ivi.com,
www.hnews@world.std.com, www.herbalgram.org, and
www.EnvPrevHealthCtrAtl.com.

The Internet has thousands of sites related to information on vitamins, minerals and herbs. Many of these sites are related to the sale of these products. Such as,

1. www.vitaz.com
2. www.twinlabs.com
3. www.naturesway.com
4. www.naturesherbs.com
5. www.natplus.com
6. www.earthrise.com
7. www.mapi.com
8. www.solgar.com

It is best to be very specific on what information you are looking for on the various subjects. Individuals who live in or close to Cincinnati, Ohio may use The Lloyd Library and Museum, which houses the world's largest collection of botanical literature.

Health Letters, Health Books, Magazines and Journals

The following list of health letters, health books, magazines and journals is very subjective and not comprehensive. Those individuals wishing additional information on the most recent studies regarding health and nutrition should visit the Internet. You may also find a vast assortment of health related books, magazines and journals with past and present research reports, by consulting with your favorite book , store, university libraries, public libraries and/or botanical museums.

Health Letters:

DEEPAK CHOPRA'S Infinite Possibilities for Body, Mind & Soul, from the Publisher of Deepak Chopra's health newsletter, Palm Coast, FL.

ENVIRONMENTAL NUTRITION, from the Publisher of Environmental Nutrition, Palm Coast, FL

HARVARD HEALTH LETTER, from the Harvard Medical School, Boston, MA.

HEALTH AFTER 50 - The Johns Hopkins Medical Letter, from the Johns Hopkins Medical Institutions, Baltimore, MD.

HEALTH NEWS, from the publishers of the New England Journal of Medicine, Waltham, MA.

HEALTH & NUTRITION LETTER, from Tufts University School of Medicine and School of Nutrition Science, Boston, MA.

MAYO CLINIC HEALTH LETTER, from the Mayo Clinic, Rochester, MN.

NUTRITION ACTION HEALTH LETTER, from the Center for Science in the Public Interest (CSPI), Washington, DC.

DR. ANDREW WEIL's - SELF HEALING, edited by Andrew Weil, MD Publisher: Thorne Communications, Inc. Morris, IL.

WELLNESS LETTER, from the University of California Berkeley, Berkeley, CA.

LIFETIME HEATH LETTER, from the University of Texas, Houston Heath Science Center, Houston, TX

Health Magazines:

AMERICAN HEALTH for Women, from the Publisher of "American Health for Women", by RD Publications, Inc., New York, NY.

HEALTH, from the Publisher of "Health Magazine", by Time, Inc. New York, NY.

MEN'S HEALTH, from the Publisher of "Men's Health Magazine", by Rodale Press, Inc. Emmaus, PA.

NATURAL HEALTH, from the Publisher of "Natural Health", by Boston Common Press Limited Partnership, Boston MA

THE NATURAL WAY, from the Publisher of "The Natural Way", by Natural Way Publications, Inc. Rye Brook, NY.

Books and Resources for Vitamins and Minerals:

Adams, Ruth. *The Complete Home Guide to all the Vitamins.* Publisher: Larchmont Books, New York, NY - 1972.

Balch, James F. MD Phyllis A Balch, C.N.C. *Prescription for Nutritional Healing.* Publisher. Avery Publishing Group, Inc., Garden City Park, New York. - 1990.

Bergner, Paul. *The Healing Power of Minerals,* Special Nutrients and Trace Elements. Publisher: Prima Publishing Co. Rocklin, CA - 1997.

Bland, Jeffrey. *Medical Applications of Clinical Nutrition.* Publisher: Keats Publishing Company, New Canaan, CT. - 1983.

Bricklin, Mark. *Practical Encyclopedia of Natural Healing.* Publisher: Rodal Press, Emmaus, PA - 1976.

Chevallier, Andrew. *The Encyclopedia of Medicinal Plants.* Publisher: D K Publishing, Inc. New York, NY. - 1996.

Dorling Kindersley Limited and The American Medical Association *Home Medical Encyclopedia.* Publisher: Random House, Inc., New York, NY. - 1989.

Eades, Mary Dan, M.D. *The Doctor's Complete Guide to Vitamins and Minerals. Publisher.* Dell Publishing Group, Inc. and The Philip Lief Group, Inc. New York, NY - 1994.

Garrison, Robert H. Jr., MA, R.Ph. and Elizabeth Somer, M.S., R.D. *The Nutrition Desk Reference.* Publisher: Keats Publishing, Inc. New Canaan, CT. - 1995.

Griffith, H. Winter. *The Complete Guide of Vitamins, Minerals, Supplements and Herbs.* Publisher: Fisher Books, Tucson, AZ. - 1988.

Hendler, Sheldon Saul, M. D., Ph.D. *The Doctor's Vitamin and Mineral Encyclopedia.* A Fireside Book. Publisher: Simon & Schuster, New York, NY. - 1991.

Lavon, J. Dunne. *Nutrition Almanac.* Third Edition, Nutrition Search, Inc., John D. Kirschmann, Director. Publisher: McGraw-Hill Publishing Company, McGraw-Hill, Inc. New York, NY. - 1990.

Lesser, Michael. *Nutrition and Vitamin Therapy.* Publisher: Grove Press, New York, NY - 1980.

Lowe, Carl. *The Complete Vitamin Book.* Publisher: The Berkley Publishing Group New York, NY. - 1994.

McDonald, Arline, Ph.D. RD, Annette Natow, Ph.D., RD and Jo-Ann Heslin, MA, RD. *The Complete Book of Vitamins & Minerals.* by the Editors of Consumer Guide, Publisher: Publications Int'l., Ltd. Lincolnwood, Illinois. - 1994.

Mindell, Earl. Earl Mindell's - *Vitamin Bible.* Publisher: Warner Books, A Times Warner Company, New York, NY. - 1991.

Mindell, Earl. Earl Mindell's - *Shaping Up with Vitamins.* Publisher: Warner Books, A Times Warner Company, New York, NY - 1985.

Netzer, Corinne T. *The Complete Book of Vitamin and Mineral Counts.* Publisher: Dell Publishing Group, Inc. New York, NY - 1997.

Null, Gary. *The Complete Guide to Health and Nutrition, A Source Book for a Healthy Life.* Publisher: Dell Publishing Group, Inc. New York, NY. - 1984.

Null, Gary and Steve Null. *The Complete Handbook of Nutrition.* Publisher: Robert Speller & Sons, New York, NY - 1972.

Passwater, Richard A. *The New Supernutrition.* Publisher: Pocket Books, New York, NY - 1991.

Pauling, Linus. *Vitamin C and the Common Cold.* Publisher: Bantam Books, New York, NY ' 1971.

Pauling, Linus. *Vitamin C and the Common Cold and the Flu.* Publisher: W. H. Freeman, New York, NY - 1976.

Prevention Magazine's *Complete Book of Vitamins and Minerals,* from the Publisher: Wings Books, Distributor: Random House Value Publishing, Inc., by arrangement with Rodale Press, Inc. Emmaus, Pa. - 1988.

Prevention Magazine's *Food and Nutrition.* Edited by Prevention Magazines Health Books. Publisher: The Berkley Publishing Group and Rodale Press, Inc. New York, NY. - 1996.

Rodale, J. I. Prevention Magazine's *The Complete Book of Minerals for Health,* Publisher: Rodale Press, Inc. Emmaus, PA - 1976 and 1981.

Rosenberg, Harold and A. N. Feldzaman. *The Doctor's Book of Vitamin Therapy:* Megavitamins for Health, Publisher: Putnam's New York, NY - 1974.

Saltman, Paul, Ph.D., Joel Gurin and Ira Mothner. *The Nutrition Book.* The University of California, San Diego. Publisher: Little, Brown & Company, New York, NY. - 1993.

Silerman, Harold M. Pharm. D., Joseph A. Romano, Pharm. D. and Gary Elmer, Ph.D. *The Vitamin Book.* Publisher: Bantam Books, New York, NY. - 1985.

The National Research Counsel. *Recommended Dietary Allowances,* (10th Edition). Publisher: National Academy of Sciences - National Research Counsel Washington, DC. - 1989.

The American Medical Association & The American Pharmaceutical Association:

The American Medical Association - Drug Evaluation Annual, Chapter 96, Vitamins and Minerals Pages: 2157 - 2179, Washington, DC. - 1994.

The American Pharmaceutical Association - Handbook of Non-prescription Drugs, Nutritional Supplements, Vitamin & Mineral Products. Washington, DC - 1993, 1994 and 1995.

Books and Resources for Herbs:

Beinfield, Harriet and Efrem Korngold. *Between Heaven and Earth,* A Guide to Chinese Medicine. Publisher: Ballantine Books, New York, NY. - 1991.

Bremness, Lesley. *The Complete Book of Herbs.* Publisher: Viking, New York, NY. - 1988.

Brown, Donald J., N. D. *Herbal Prescriptions for Better Health, Your Up-To-Date Guide to the Most Effective Herbal Treatments.* Publisher: Prima Communications, Inc. - 1996.

Castleman, Michael. *The Healing Herbs - The Ultimate Guide to the Curative Power of Nature's Medicines.* Publisher: Bantam Books, a division of Bantam Doubleday Dell Publishing Group, Inc. New York, NY. - 1995.

Crellin, John K. and Jane Philpott. *Herbal Medicine, Past and Present,* Volume 2. A Reference Guide to Medicinal Plants. Publisher: Duke University Press, Durham, NC. - 1990.

Culpeper, Nicholas. *Culpeper's Complete Herbal.* Publisher: W. Foulsham & Co., Ltd., London, England. - 1987.

Cumston, Charles Greene. *An Introduction to the History of Medicine.* Publisher: Dorset Press, New York, NY. - 1987.

Duke, James A. *Handbook of Medicinal Herbs.* Publisher: CRC Press, Pleasantville, NY. - 1985.

Elias, Jason M.A., L.Ac. and Shelagh Ryan Masline. *The A to Z Guide to Healing Herbal Remedies.* Publisher: Wings Books, Random House Value Publishing, Inc. New York, NY - 1996.

Fulder, Stephen. *Ginseng - Magical Herb of the East.* Publisher: Thorsons Publishing, Northamptonshire, England. - 1988.

Harris, Lloyd J. *The Book of Garlic.* Publisher: Aris Books, Berkeley, CA. - 1979.

Heinerman, John Ph.D. *The Healing Benefits of Garlic.* Publisher: Wings Books, New York, NY. - 1994.

Hoffmann, David. *The Complete Illustrated Holistic Herbal, A Safe and Practical Guide to Making and Using Herbal Remedies.* Publisher: Element Books, Inc. Rockport, MA. - 1996.

Hoffman, D. *The Herbal Handbook, A User's Guide to Medical Herbalism.* Publisher: Healing Arts Press, Rochester, VT. - 1988.

Hyatt, Richard. *Chinese Herbal Medicine.* Publisher: Schocken Books, New York, NY. - 1978.

Kessler, David, M. D. with Sheila Buff. *The Doctor's Complete Guide to Healing Herbs.* Produced by The Philip Lief Group, Inc. Publisher: The Berkley Publishing Group New York, NY. - 1996.

Kowalchik, Claire and William H Hylton. *Rodales Illustrated Encyclopedia of Herbs.* Publisher: Rodale Press, Inc. Emmaus, PA. - 1987.

Landis, Robyn. *The Herbal Defense.* Publisher: Warner Books, Inc. New York, NY - 1997.

Lust, John. *The Herb Book.* Publisher: Bantam Books, New York, NY. - 1974.

Mindell, Earl. Earl Mindell's - *HERB BIBLE.* A Fireside Book, Publisher: Simon & Schuster, New York, NY. - 1992.

Murray, Michael T. N.D. and Joseph Pizzorno N.D. *Encyclopedia of Natural Medicine.* Publisher: Prima Publishing Company. - 1990.

Murray, Michael T., N.D. *Natural Alternatives to Over-the-Counter and Prescription Drugs.* Publisher: William Morrow. - 1994.

Ody, Penelope. *The Complete Medicinal Herbal - A Practical Guide to the Healing Properties of Herbs.* Publisher: Dorling Kindersley, Inc. New York, NY. - 1993.

Reid, Daniel. *Chinese Herbal Medicine.* Publisher: Shambhala, Boston, MA. - 1987.

Ryman, Daniele. *Aromatherapy, The Complete Guide to Plant and Flower Essences for Health and Beauty.* Publisher: Bantam Books, New York, NY. - 1993.

Peterson, Nicole. *Culpeper's Guide, Herbs and Health.* Publisher: Webb & Bower, London, England. - 1989.

Siraisi, Nancy. *Medieval and Early Renaissance Medicine.* Publisher: University Press, Chicago, IL. - 1990.

Stansbury, Jill, N. D. *Herbs for Health and Healing, A Wellness Guide to Herbal Remedies.* Publisher: Publications International, Ltd. - 1997.

Smith, F. Porter and G. A. Stuart. *Chinese Medicinal Herbs.* Publisher: Georgetown Press, San Francisco, CA. - 1973.

Stuart, Malcolm, Edited by. *The Encyclopedia of Herbs and Herbalism.* Publisher: Grosset & Dunlap, New York, NY. - 1979.

Stuckey, Maggie. *The Complete Herb Book.* Produced by The Philip Lief Group, Inc. Publisher: The Berkley Publishing Group, New York, NY. - 1994.

Tierra, Michael. *Planetary Herbology.* Publisher: Lotus Press, Santa Fe, NM. - 1988.

Tisserand, Robert. *Aromatherapy, To Heal and Tend the Body.* Publisher: Lotus Press, Santa Fe, NM. - 1988.

Weil, Andrew. *Natural Health, Natural Medicine.* Publisher: Houghton Mifflin Co. New York, NY - 1995.

Weil, Andrew. *Health and Healing.* Publisher: Houghton Mifflin Co. New York, NY - 1995.

Weil, Andrew. *Whole Earth Review - 64, A New Look at Botanical Medicine* Publisher: Houghton Mifflin Co. New York, NY - 1989.

Wheelwright, Edith Grey. *Medicinal Plants and Their History.* Publisher: Progressive Publishing, - 1988.

Journals and News Letters for Natural Products:

The American Journal of Chinese Medicine, article by Petkov, V. D. * A. H. Mosharrof, - 1987. Article by M. Yamamoto, - 1983. Article by I. M. Popov and W. J. Goldwag - 1973.

American Journal of Clinical Nutrition, article(s) by A. K. Bordia - 1981. Article by R. C. Jain - 1975 & 1977. Article by L. S. Tong - 1980. Growth and Development - Zinc Supplementation, Vol. 63, No. 4, April 1996. Vitamin and Mineral Status in Physically Active Men, January 1992.

American Journal of Public Health, article by Kim I. Williamson, Vitamin & Mineral Supplement Use and Mortality in a US Cohort, April 1993.

Canadian Pharmaceutical Journal, article by D. V. C. Awang - 1989. Article by R. F Chandler - 1985.

Drugs of the Future, article by P. Braquet - 1987.

Food and Cosmetic Toxicology, article(s) by D. L. Opdyke - 1975.

Health Food Business, Aloe Vera: "Reversed, Mysterious Healer." by Timothy R. Fox - December 1990.

HerbalGram, article by C. Hobbs, Editor: Mark Blumenthal, Austin TX - 1989. Reference was made to many other *HerbalGram* Newsletters and has been a very valuable source of information since 1983.

International Journal of Sport Nutrition, article by Sobal J. Marquart, Vitamin & Mineral Supplement Use Among Athletes, December 1994. Journal of the American College of Nutrition, article by T. L. Bazzarre, Vitamin and Mineral Supplement Use and Nutritional Status of Athletes, April 1993.

Journal of the American Dietetic Association, 96 (1) 73 - 7. January 1996

Journal of the American Medical Association, article by R. K. Siegel - 1979. Article by T. J. Chamberlin - 1970. Article by J. W. Conn - 1968. Article by J. R. Lewis - 1974.

Journal of the American Medical Technology, article by J. P. Haggers - 1979.

Journal of Biosocial Sciences, The Turlock Vitamin and Mineral Supplement Trial, E. Peritz, April 1994.

Journal of Natural Products, article by G. Kupchan and S. Karmin - 1976. Article by K. Michinori - 1981. Article by Y. Oshima & K. Sato - 1987. Article by L. A. Mitscher - 1980.

The Journal of Nutrition and The Journal of Nutritional Biochemistry, information from various articles and notes were used from these Journals, from 1992.

Journal of New Chinese Medicine, article by L. P. Cai - 1984.

The Lancet, is a journal providing valuable sources of information on herbs and a variety of remedies from a number of issues from 1981 to 1988.

New England Journal of Medicine, article by C. R. Dorso - 1980. Article by J. D. Blachley & J. P. Knochel - 1980. Article by F. Lai - 1980.

The New York Times, article by J. N. Wilford - March 1988. And an article by Jane E. Brody, February 15, 1990.

Nutrition Research, article by B. H. S. Lau - 1987.

Reader's Digest Magic and Medicine of Plants. Publisher: Reader's Digest Books, Pleasantville, NY. - 1986.

World Review of Nutrition and Dietetics, article by S. M. Zifferblatt, Nutrition and Fitness Recommendations, when Science is in Transition, Vitamin and Mineral Supplementation, 72:177-89, 1993.

Figure and Chart References:

Figure 1: *Adapted from "Dietary Goals for the United States"*, 2nd ed. Select Committee on Nutrition and Human Needs, United States Senate. Washington, DC: US Government Printing Office, 1977, Page 5.

Figure 2. Adapted from Travis, S and Fry B. "*Energy: Our Food and Our Needs*", Ithica, NY: Division of Nutritional Sciences, Cornell University.

Figure 3. Adapted and modified from the book by Robinson, C. H., *Normal and Therapeutic Nutrition.* Publisher: Macmillan Publishing Co. New York, NY 1972.